Making Sense of Spirituality in Nursing and Health Care Practice

of related interest

Ageing, Disability and Spirituality
Addressing the Challenge of Disability in Later Life
Edited by Elizabeth MacKinlay
ISBN 978 1 84310 584 8

Children and Spirituality
Searching for Meaning and Connectedness
Brendan Hyde
ISBN 978 1 84310 589 3

The Spiritual Dimension of Childhood
Kate Adams, Brendan Hyde and Richard Woolley
ISBN 978 1 84310 602 9

Prayer in Counselling and Psychotherapy
Exploring a Hidden Meaningful Dimension
Peter Madsen Gubi
Foreword by Brian Thorne
ISBN 978 1 84310 519 0

Spirituality, Ethics and Care
Simon Robinson
ISBN 978 1 84310 498 8

The Spirit of the Child
Revised Edition
David Hay
With Rebecca Nye
ISBN 978 1 84310 371 4

Talking About Spirituality in Health Care Practice
A Resource for the Multi-Professional Health Care Team
Gillian White
ISBN 978 1 84310 305 9

Spiritual Growth and Care in the Fourth Age of Life
Elizabeth MacKinlay
ISBN 978 1 84310 231 1

Spirituality in Health Care Contexts
Edited by Helen Orchard
ISBN 978 1 85302 969 1

Making Sense of Spirituality in Nursing and Health Care Practice

An Interactive Approach

Second Edition

Wilfred McSherry

Foreword by Keith Cash

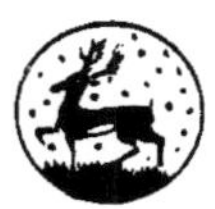

Jessica Kingsley Publishers
London and Philadelphia

Figures 2.3 and 3.2 are adapted from Stoll, R.I (1989) 'The essence of spirituality' in V.B. Carson, *Spiritual Dimensions of Nursing Practice.* Philadelphia: WB Saunders. Reproduced with permission from Elsevier Inc.

Figure 3.3 is reproduced from Beland, I.L and Passos, J.Y. (1975) *Clinical Nursing, Third Edition.* © 1975 Macmillan Publishing Company. Reprinted with the permission of Scribner, a division of Simon and Schuster.

Box 4.1 is reproduced from Nyatanga, B. and Astley-Pepper, M. (2005) *Hidden Aspects of Palliative Care.* London: Quay Books. Reproduced with permission from Quay Books.

First published in 2006
by Jessica Kingsley Publishers
116 Pentonville Road
London N1 9JB, UK
and
400 Market Street, Suite 400
Philadelphia, PA 19106, USA

www.jkp.com

Copyright © Wilfred McSherry 2006
Foreword copyright © Keith Cash 2006

Printed digitally since 2008

The right of Wilfred McSherry to be identified as author of this work has been asserted by him in accordance with the Copyright, Designs and Patents Act 1988.

All rights reserved. No part of this publication may be reproduced in any material form (including photocopying or storing it in any medium by electronic means and whether or not transiently or incidentally to some other use of this publication) without the written permission of the copyright owner except in accordance with the provisions of the Copyright, Designs and Patents Act 1988 or under the terms of a licence issued by the Copyright Licensing Agency Ltd, Saffron House, 6–10 Kirby Street, London EC1N 8TS. Applications for the copyright owner's written permission to reproduce any part of this publication should be addressed to the publisher.

Warning: The doing of an unauthorised act in relation to a copyright work may result in both a civil claim for damages and criminal prosecution.

Library of Congress Cataloging in Publication Data

McSherry, Wilfred.

Making sense of spirituality in nursing and health care practice : an interactive approach / Wilfred McSherry ; foreword by Keith Cash. -- 2nd ed.

p. cm.

Includes bibliographical references and indexes.

ISBN-13: 978-1-84985-265-4 (pbk. : alk. paper)

ISBN-10: 1-84985-265-0 (pbk. : alk. paper) 1. Holistic nursing--Religious aspects. 2. Holistic nursing--Moral and ethical aspects. 3. Spirituality. I. Title.

RT85.2.M37 2006

610.73--dc22

2006013531

British Library Cataloguing in Publication Data

A CIP catalogue record for this book is available from the British Library

ISBN 978 1 84985 265 4

I dedicate this second edition of *Making Sense of Spirituality in Nursing and Health Care Practice* to my deceased parents, Dorothy and Wilfred McSherry.

Acknowledgements

I would like to take this opportunity to thank all those people who have supported and inspired me to pursue my interests in the spiritual dimension. First, I would like to thank my family and friends whose words of encouragement and love have provided continual support and presence. Secondly, I would like to thank my PhD supervisors Professor Keith Cash, Professor Alan White and Dr Linda Ross for refining my thinking and understanding, challenging me to explore more fully the depths of spirituality. Without their guidance, wisdom and encouragement I do not think I would have completed the journey. Deep appreciation to all the people who have participated in my research investigation, their views and words have shaped and moulded my perceptions of spirituality and spiritual care. Thirdly, I would like to thank Jessica Kingsley Publishers for publishing this second edition and Professor John Swinton series editor for his constructive comments.

Contents

Foreword

Why should a book on spirituality in health care be published, and why should it reach a second edition like this book? The fact that there is a demand for a second edition of this book seems to indicate that there is a need for it. But why should health professionals concern themselves with a concept like spirituality? This depends, of course, on how one sees health care. There is a fashion now to talk about more holistic care, although health services still tend to be dominated by the disease and curative models of health. The problem with holism is trying to define what the whole is. Where does one stop when considering a person and the way that they construct their health? Health includes so many different aspects of the person – it is not just their anatomy and physiology, but also their relationships with other people, institutions and society, as well as their personal sense of well-being.

Perhaps one way out of the problem of holism is to look at what makes us human. On the one hand, there are universals that make us human, on the other the differences between us in the ways that we make sense of the world. We all need to eat, to have shelter, to reproduce and to make sense of the world. But how we do these things can vary from individual to individual and community to community. Taking account of spirituality therefore not only recognizes it as one of the things that is important to us as human beings, but also recognises the differences in the ways that people interpret the spiritual.

Illness presents a threat to the identity of an individual as well as impacting on the quality of their life. The use of medical terms like HIV, schizophrenia, and epilepsy, as well as descriptive terms like obesity, carry a whole range of meanings that imply a moral judgement on a person's will-power, strength of character, physical attractiveness or social responsibility. Health care is an intensely moral activity. All the decisions taken by health professionals have implications for well being, justice and care and therefore for the personal identity of the person being cared for. As the Western model of medicine spreads across the globe, the issue becomes more pressing. There is a paradox in this process of globalization – with globalization comes the fragmentation of traditional sources of meaning for people's lives, but also a strengthening of them in some areas. The decline of orthodox religion in the West is paralleled by a growth in the developing world. In the West there is a heady cocktail of different approaches to faith, some institutional, some individual. The health professional cannot expect to be an expert in all the ways in which people make sense of the world and their illnesses. But what can be expected is that they are sensitive to the existence of these multiple ways of interpreting the world and do not ignore them when they are caring for people.

This book has already made an excellent contribution to sensitizing health care professionals to the importance of spirituality as a factor in what makes us human, and its importance in delivering humane health care. I am sure that the second edition will continue this important work.

Professor Keith Cash
Memorial University, Newfoundland, Canada
and WHO Consultant, Damascus, Syria

Preface to the second edition

The practice of health care is dynamic, continually evolving with new knowledge and insight gained in terms of disease processes, treatments and care management. Furthermore, contemporary health care faces new challenges with greater emphasis placed on such things as professional accountability, inter-professional working, evidence-based and anti-discriminatory practice, and the ever-growing demands of a public who are informed of their rights and acutely aware of what standards of care they should receive. In addition, the threat of litigation is all too real and the importance of good documentation is constantly being drummed home.

This litany of contemporary issues seems rather pessimistic in that it presents a picture of health care that is bureaucratic, constraining, oppressive, and divisive in setting up an us (health care professionals) and them (patient, clients, consumers) mentality rather than partnership working. It also highlights that maybe one of the reasons why this negative culture prevails is the demise of the 'essence of care' within our health care system and society – we are constantly hearing politicians and social commentators stressing that there is a loss of respect. The constant need to satisfy a bureaucratic (political) agenda and to persistently safeguard one's own professional integrity may have resulted in a preoccupation with 'self'; this perspective could also be extended to include fixation with the material and the secular. This view seems to prevail despite research suggesting the contrary – that societies and individuals thirst for and are actively seeking a spiritual dimension (Hay and Hunt 2000; Heelas and Woodhead 2005).

This contradiction, that individuals are seeking to be spiritual while becoming increasingly egotistical, whether this is us satisfying our own financial and political ends or professionally setting boundaries and becoming very territorial in how we work, is perplexing. However, we must not forget that all individuals have the potential towards goodness, and this has certainly been witnessed and expressed in recent natural disasters and other catastrophic events that have shaken the fabric of societies and the modern world. Wright (2002, p.24) tells us that 'Ground zero' may have accelerated people turning away from materialistic lifestyles towards personal spiritual well-being.

The human spirit is continually being expressed in the way that people working in health care constantly sacrifice themselves in the service of those in need. Yet, despite overwhelming generosity, societies, cultures and professions can create and harbour individuals who are intent on harming fellow citizens in the advancement of their own or a greater extremist cause. These imbalances, extremes and contradictions within society are also evident within health care practice, but thankfully they do not manifest themselves so frequently. We have a health care system that asserts the mantras of 'holism' and 'spiritual care', presenting the individual as an elaborate blend of physical, psychological, social, spiritual and environmental needs while operating in a system and organizations that are becoming highly specialist, technological and reductionist in their approach. It could also be said that the central tenet 'care' has been eroded as individuals are described either as providers or as consumers; we are witnessing a depersonalisation of care and the carer.

The economic constraint placed on many health care professionals has resulted in the devolution of skills to individuals who are perhaps not appropriately qualified. Moreover, a disproportionate amount of time seems to be spent on administrative duties, at the expense of listening to and working alongside patients and service users. Needless to say, many health care professionals feel dissatisfied and disgruntled in their present roles. The net effect is a health care system that appears to have lost its way in terms of 'caring' for both the cared and the carer. This view is certainly evident in the writings of many health care professionals. For example, Harold G. Koenig (2001, p.33), one of the most prominent researchers and writers into the area of religion and spirituality, states:

> In recent times, I have heard more and more patients express dissatisfaction with medical care and more and more physicians indicate that their job has become less fulfilling. I believe that physicians and patients may be responding to how mechanistic the practice of medicine has become. Bringing spirituality back into medicine may be what we all need.

At the heart of holistic health care, and arguably good health care practice, is spirituality – a concept that throughout its long history and association with health care has never witnessed and enjoyed such popularity as it does today. One only needs to look at the vast number of books published on the subject within health care to gauge the strength of this revival. Yet, despite this growing popularity, research still suggests that many people working within health care, professional and 'non-professional', are still struggling to understand the concept or, more importantly, they are not aware of this dimension within themselves, their patients, clients or the communities they serve.

This lack of awareness is not a signal for all the converted, academics and practitioners to proselytize the uninitiated to the spiritual dimension. On the contrary, a lack of awareness, or unfamiliarity with the language of spirituality, does not necessarily mean that the spiritual needs of patients, clients and staff are being unmet. With this point in mind, I would like to present again a paragraph from the preface of the first edition because it still has poignancy and relevance today:

> I am conscious that some of the material presented reflects a Judeo-Christian approach to spirituality. However, this is not a deliberate attempt to exclude other world faiths but is a reflection of my personal experiences. I hope that readers from other world faiths will still find the material relevant, stimulating and challenging. With reference to the concepts of spirituality and spiritual need, these terms may not be universally understood or relevant to all individuals. It would be a grave mistake to assume that everyone who requires health care will present with spiritual needs or identify with the concepts discussed. (McSherry 2000, pp.ix–x)

Despite a great deal of academic, political and professional activity in raising the profiles of spirituality and spiritual care, research suggests that many health care professionals still feel inadequately prepared to deal with the spiritual needs of their patients or service users and are asking for more attention to be accredited to this dimension within educational programmes.

With all the aforementioned contemporary constraints and developments, I felt that there was a need to bring my book up to date and produce a second edition. This new edition has been updated where appropriate in terms of literature, drawing on some of the modern thinking and research on spirituality in health care. However, I have not been overly radical in that I have maintained the general style, structure, content and features of the first edition. The rationale for this is that a wide range of students and health care professionals felt that this was an accessible and successful introduction to the subject. The phrase, 'Why fix something if it isn't broken', comes to mind.

One key difference is that I have attempted to be inclusive, writing a generic text for all health care professions, rather than focusing exclusively upon nursing. The justification for this change in focus was that several individuals from a range of health care professions contacted me – for example, social work, chaplaincy and counselling, stressing how beneficial they had found the book, despite the nursing focus. They felt the material was valuable because the content and the principles being advocated were generic, having meaning and relevance for all health care professions, and people working in diverse care settings. Therefore, I hope that readers will continue to find this revised edition useful, and that it will assist in enhancing their understanding of spirituality and spiritual care, and in highlighting the importance of this dimension to health care practice at both a personal and practical level. I hope that the reflective exercise and activities will continue to engage and enable readers to make sense of the challenges and difficulties that they face in providing spiritual health care under sometimes difficult and often adverse circumstances.

Wilfred McSherry

References

Hay, D. and Hunt, K. (2000) Understanding the Spirituality of People who Don't go to Church. A report on the findings of the Adults' Spirituality project at the University of Nottingham.

Heelas, P. and Woodhead, L. (2005) *The Spiritual Revolution.* Oxford: Blackwell Publishing.

Koenig, H.G. (2001) 'Spiritual assessment in medical practice.' *American Family Physician 63*, 1, 30, 33.

McSherry, W. (2000) *Making Sense of Spirituality in Nursing Practice: An Interactive Approach.* Edinburgh: Churchill Livingstone.

Wright, S. (2002) 'Out of the ashes.' *Nursing Standard 16*, 24, 24.

1

Spiritual Heritage of Health Care

Introduction

A study of the historical development of health care reveals that it has a deep rich religious or what could be classified as a 'spiritual heritage'. Culliford (2002, p.1434) writes: 'Medicine, once fully bound up with religion, retains a sacred dimension for many.' It could be argued that health care within many modern societies emerged out of the ethos of the Judeo-Christian principle of charity – caring for those who were less fortunate than oneself or out of a greater humanitarian need to help one's fellow man, woman. This chapter provides a brief exploration of health care's historical heritage, indicating that religion and to a lesser degree spirituality has always been present, whether or not there has been a conscious realization of this by contemporary health care theorists. This chapter also introduces some of the growing debate surrounding the effect that technological and medical advancement may have upon the relationship between spirituality and health care practice.

Activity 1.1

Before proceeding with this chapter spend several minutes reflecting upon images associated with the term 'health care professional' (I have chosen 'nurse' because this is my profession); however, you might want to reflect upon your own profession be it medicine, social work, chaplaincy, radiography, operating department assistant, occupational therapy, etc. Write down any words, thoughts or ideas that come to mind. Pay particular attention to some of the images in general use associated with your group – for example, in my discipline 'angel of mercy' – or you may want to reflect upon some of the qualities or virtues that are generic to all health care professions such as patience and kindness.

Symbols and signs

Your reflections may have revealed several terms, phrases or images associated with health care professionals whether this be nursing or your chosen profession (Box 1.1). Some of these may be historical in origin, indicating specific virtues such as patience, kindness or selfless dedication, while others may be related to garments of clothing such as uniforms or hats (for example, in nursing remnants of the nun's habit and wimple). Modern interpretations may represent comedy as seen on seaside postcards, or the archetypal matron personified by Hatty Jacques, or even an object of desire as represented in the *Carry On* films by Barbara Windsor. In recent years, there may also be some negativity surrounding specific professional groups. For example, public perception towards medicine has undoubtedly been influenced by the actions and scandals of specific individuals (doctors), bringing to mind the crimes of Harold Shipman which led to the Shipman Inquiry conducted by Dame Janet Smith, whose final report was published in January 2005 (The Shipman Inquiry 2001, www.the-shipman-inquiry.org) and, in social work, the Victoria Climbié Inquiry undertaken by Lord Laming, whose report was published in 2003 (Cm 5730). These cases seem to have eroded public confidence and shattered the caring and trusting views held by many towards medicine and social work. Equally, these cases highlight the importance of all health care professions and social and welfare agencies working collaboratively in providing care. Such events have undoubtedly left a legacy in terms of public opinion leading to reviews as to how some health care professionals are educated and their practice monitored.

By examining both the historical and modern images of health care, it is evident that there has been a dramatic shift in how health care professionals are perceived and portrayed in many Western and Eastern societies. The historical image of health care professionals being morally virtuous has been replaced sadly by images of mistrust, in some instances fuelled by comedy in

Box 1.1 Historical and modern images associated with nursing

Historical

Symbol of virtues, kindness, caring

An angel of mercy

Uniform – remnant of the nun's habit

Selflessness, vocation

Modern

Comedy – *Carry On* films, postcards, Channel 4

Barbara Windsor – object of desire, envy, lust

Archetypal matron – control subordination to medical profession

Financial remuneration – career for life

the mass media, which present doctors as cold-hearted and focusing purely on the physical, whereas nurses seem to be presented as objects of desire and ridicule – for example, the programme titled *Nurses* on Channel 4. Other professional groups seem immune to ridicule because they are not portrayed frequently in the mass media. It would appear that respect for the sacred and spiritual values inherent in health care have been decayed. A possible explanation for this may be found in how the spiritual heritage of health care is being eroded and replaced by modern, secular, material values. It is suggested that there is a subconscious attempt by Western society to distance health care from its past association with formal religious values and principles. This approach seems very negative and perhaps not representative of all sections in society. However, some of the negative attitudes projected towards health care are continuing to be challenged by television programmes that seek to portray health care professionals in a more 'professional' manner – for example, *Casualty*, *Holby City* and the *Golden Hour* on British television and *ER* across the Atlantic. The remainder of this chapter will address some of these issues in more detail.

Historical and modern developments

A review of the literature addressing the spiritual dimension reveals that indeed many of the health care professions arise out of a strong historical association with religious and spiritual traditions (Cobb and Robshaw 1998; Cook 2004; Narayanasamy 2001; Rumbold 2002; Whipp 1998). Indeed, Smart (1969, p.10) argues that to understand the developments of any society one must first gain insight into the religions that are found within it:

> To understand human history and human life it is necessary to understand religion, and in the contemporary world one must understand other nations' ideologies and faith in order to grasp the meaning of life as seen from perspectives often very different from our own.

Therefore, when exploring the spiritual heritage of health care, there is a fundamental need to become aware of the religious influences that have shaped and guided health care throughout history. This point is crucial in contemporary society where there is now vast ethnic, racial and cultural diversity. It is imperative that the voices of all groups in a pluralistic society inform any debate on spirituality in health care. The need to engage with and reflect the beliefs and needs of all sections of society is recognized in many of the texts written on spirituality – for example, see Markham (1998), Narayanasamy (2001), Orchard (2001). The outcome of Activity 1.1 reveals that health care does have a strong formal religious and spiritual legacy that has influenced both the individual's and society's perceptions; however, this legacy is perhaps mono-cultural in that it reflects Western religious thought. The activity also indicates that some secular values and interpretations are replacing this rich religious/spiritual heritage.

The strong association between mind, body and spirit or soul was recognized by ancient civilizations. This is reflected in, for example, the 'Hippocratic Oath' taken by many medical students upon graduation which in the modern version states, 'I will remember that there is art to medicine as well as science, and that warmth, sympathy, and understanding may outweigh the surgeon's knife or the chemist's drug' (Lasagna 1964). Despite some criticism of the 'Hippocratic Oath', the virtues it espouses and the recognition that health care is an intricate blend of art and science have become central to the delivery of all health care practice.

In many Western and Eastern societies, an imbalance in the spirit was believed to manifest itself through physical illness, disease, demonic possession or madness (Holland and Hogg 2001; Narayanasamy 1999). During the Middle Ages, people in Western countries perceived the outbreak of disease or the presence of an illness as a punishment from God. People's experience of the physical, material world was intimately linked with the awareness of a higher power that controlled the individual's internal and external world, maintaining equilibrium and restoring order when chaos prevailed.

Tripartite being

Robbins (1991) suggests that the human is a tripartite being composed of mind, body and spirit. Although this illustration is divisive in that it fragments the individual, the analogy does indicate that the spiritual element must be in harmony with the physical and mental for spiritual development to occur. This realization of the importance of the spiritual dimension is reinforced in many religious teachings. It is not possible to provide an insight into the teachings of all world religions; here a brief overview of the Judeo-Christian approach is offered.

Awareness of a higher power

In the Old Testament, the people of Israel awaited deliverance from their suffering and oppression. While in exile and journeying to the Promised Land, their God rescued and delivered them from the hands of their captors. A higher authority had intervened in the destiny of humankind, restoring order and providing a template or code of living that governed and guided the beliefs, values and behaviours of the Jewish people. This awareness of a higher power or divine being intervening in creation and controlling environmental, social, and individual destiny was not just specific to the Judeo-Christian tradition. Historically, people have worshipped or offered sacrifices to the elements, fire, rain, sun and beasts in an attempt to improve their prosperity, indeed their chance of survival. Cupitt (1995, p.90) writes: 'The god may previously have been a tribal totem or clan divinity in animal form or a fertility figure…'

The realization that a higher authority may control the destiny of humankind resulted in the emergence of different religions and cultures, all with their own forms of expression, beliefs, rituals and guiding principles. Carson (1989) and Bradshaw (1994) reveal how my profession, nursing, has been steeped and fashioned by Christianity, a view shared by Ellis (1980, p.42):

> Did not nursing historically develop in a religious milieu in which love of God and mankind was expressed through care, compassion, and charity, to the sick, the poor, the orphans and the outcasts.

If one examines Ellis' quotation, then implicit within it is the notion of the Christian Beatitudes. It would appear that nursing (and health care) in Western society has been profoundly influenced by the teachings of Jesus Christ, whose values have shaped and guided many societies.

Carson (1989) presents an historical overview of the development of nursing which I feel has relevance for many health care professions, since it is not implausible to suggest that some health care professions have their origins from within nursing. She describes one of the most famous of the religious orders, The Knights of Hospitallers of St John, who were responsible for establishing nursing and drew their members from crusaders, monks and religious brothers. This order was founded in the Middle Ages to provide nursing care for the victims of the crusades. Originally, the order was located in Jerusalem but the congregation soon spread throughout the Western world, providing nursing and spiritual care for the sick and dying.

Modernism and secularism

From the argument presented so far, you have probably deduced that we are living in an age that is dominated by things that are material and tangible, and where individuals want immediate results and rewards. Watson (1996, p.39), recognizing the erosion of the spiritual dimension from the heart of nursing, and that this could be extended to include the whole of health care, writes:

> May this era between centuries be the turning-point whereby nursing restores and further develops its caring-healing art and spiritual dimensions lest the profession collectively dies of a broken heart.

Watson warns that the spiritual dimension is the most important dimension of nursing in that it provides life to all other aspects of the profession. If health care fails to restore the spiritual dimension to its central position, then it is in danger of being replaced by something dehumanizing and cold. Within the health care literature, the terms 'modernism' and 'secularism' are used with growing regularity. However, what do these words mean? Moreover, what are the implications of them upon the spiritual dimension of health care?

If we focus upon our own existence and the things that are important to us, it is apparent that there are certain material things in life that are needed for survival such as food, shelter, warmth and water. Deprived of these important elements, we would die. Therefore, by our very physical nature we are dependent upon material things. When the words modernism, materialistic and secular are used in health care, they are often used negatively to suggest that there is a preoccupation with or over-reliance upon them at the expense of other aspects such as the spiritual dimension. Narayanasamy (1997) proposes that the spiritual aspects of individuals will receive less attention in societies that are preoccupied with technological and scientific advancements, and where individuals want immediate result or reward.

Modernism, materialism and secularism are the three main 'isms' that, in their extreme, seem to be incompatible with the notion of spirituality (Box 1.2). It is the emergence and subsequent preoccupation with these terms within health care that have resulted in the demise of the spiritual heritage. Moreover, additional forms of extremism are the notion and misconceptions that spirituality equates only with formal, institutional religion, to which many individuals attach little importance, and the danger of making stereotyped assumptions about religious minority groups (Burnard 1988; Gilliat-Ray 2001; Narayanasamy 2001).

Box 1.2 The three main 'isms'

Modernism

The term used to describe an over-preoccupation with modern technological, medical, scientific advancement.

Secularism

The belief that religious, spiritual principles have been made redundant within modern cultures.

Materialism

An over-reliance with material objects and possessions at the expense of recognizing the transcendent, mysterious aspects of human existence.

Scientific and technological advancement

If one thinks of the recent developments within health care, in particular medical and surgical practices, then one cannot be surprised that these developments and innovations have changed the way in which society perceives health care. These changes are summed up by Donley (1991, p.178): 'Today, people expect that their diseased organs will be replaced and that disability and death will be postponed.'

The innovations in scientific and medical technology mean health care has become more complex and complicated. There has also been a tremendous change in patient expectation, with individuals being more aware of their rights, challenging decisions and treatments. It would appear that the art and science of 'medicalization' still dominate and guide practice while the spiritual dimension has been relegated from the premier league to the second division. Science is still the predominant force guiding practice and shaping the direction and future of health care. Bradshaw (1996a, p.61) alerts the scientific community to the hidden dangers in following this path:

> It is not surprising that there should be a distrust of science as dehumanising and impersonal, mechanical, hard and cold. And certainly among nursing writers today, it is easy to trace a distrust with western science and what is called the biomedical.

Activity 1.2

Read the above quotation several times and see if you can think of any of your own examples from practice that may support the points that Bradshaw is making.

When reflecting upon the quotation, it is easy to identify and recall examples from your own practice that confirm Bradshaw's apprehensions. How often does one still hear the phrase, 'The appendicectomy in bed three', or, more recently, 'The lap chole (laparoscopic cholecystectomy) in bed four', the 'CABPG (coronary artery bypass graft) in bed five' or the 'stroke' or 'CVA (cerebrovascular accident) in bed six', depending upon the specialty? This attitude towards individuals reflects the cold, dehumanizing face of science and a medical model that is not holistic, individualized or patient-centred.

Kearney (1994) and Bradshaw (1996a) suggest that science, religion and the spiritual realm are all seeking answers concerning the nature and mystery of our everyday life. Therefore, science and spirituality, instead of being in opposition, should be seen as different sides of the same coin that are closely united in seeking to find out the truths about our very existence and human condition. Sloan *et al.* (1999, p.664) highlight the complex and often fraught relationship religion and science share:

> Religion and science share a complex history as well as a complex present. At various times worldwide, medical and spiritual care was dispensed by the same person. At other times, passionate, (even violent) conflicts characterized the association between religion, and medicine and science.

It may be that divisions arise because science and spirituality use different methods of enquiry to find out about the nature and structure of individuals. Science seeks to clarify by rigid control, producing evidence from experiments and trials, while spirituality is concerned with the 'touchy feely' aspects of our being that are often very mysterious and hard to pin down. It would appear that the argument that there is no place for spirituality within the scientific community is redundant, short-sighted and misguided, since spirituality and science can work in harmony answering questions about our physical and existential world.

Demise of spirituality

The health care literature implies that there has been a gradual demise of the spiritual dimension in the last years of the 20th century. Some contemporary writers on spirituality suggest that the traditional view of health care, in which spirituality was fundamental, has been replaced by a modern – 'fashionable' – approach. Bradshaw (1993, p.3) writes:

> The long held Judeo-Christian, ethical tradition of caring for the sick as an altruistic calling was now seen as archaic, irrelevant and even a dangerous myth that needed dispelling – the opiate of oppressed nurses.

Bradshaw implies that many of nursing's (this position could be extend to all working in health care) historical and spiritual traditions have changed with advances in science and medicine. These changes contradict what several prominent 20th-century nurse theorists have written about holism and individualism (Henderson 1966; Orem 1985; Peplau 1952). Tournier (1954) suggested that there is a need for physicians to focus their interventions and treatments upon the patient rather than just the illness. Tournier (1954, p.13) writes: 'We may say, then, that every illness calls for two diagnoses: one scientific, nosological and causal, and the other spiritual, a diagnosis of its meaning and purpose.' Tournier had identified the need to treat both sides of the coin (scientific and spiritual), identifying and advocating holistic care. This position was quite unprecedented in that a physician had recognized how the scientific and the spiritual could be used to manage and treat the 'whole person' (Tournier 1973).

Activity 1.3

Spend some time reflecting upon the content of the chapter so far. Make a list of possible explanations why many of the traditional and sacred values inherent in health care have been eroded.

In the course of your reflection, you may have identified several important reasons why the traditional values within health care have been replaced. Some of these reasons may be associated with issues already discussed such as scientific and technological advancement, while others may be associated with changes in the way society views spirituality.

Dawson (1945) argued that since the Renaissance, a time of enlightenment, scientific growth and discovery of the natural world, Western cultures have abandoned their religious heritage. Dawson (1945, p.249) writes:

> We have come to take it for granted that the unifying force in society is material interest, and that spiritual conviction is a source of strife and division. Modern civilization has pushed religion and the spiritual elements in culture out of the main stream of its development, so that they have lost touch with life and have become sectarianized and impoverished.

Dawson suggests that society's preoccupation with the temporal pervaded the philosophies of the medical profession and, more recently, nursing. Already in this chapter the dangers associated with the medical and surgical advances have been presented. The 20th century has seen the development and rapid institution of the medical model (Swaffield 1988).

Female subordination

Another possible reason for the erosion of the spiritual heritage of health care may be found in the authority and position that women held in society. It could be argued that many health care tasks involving caring such as nursing, were inadvertently led into adopting a divisive medical model that sought to exclude the spiritual dimension because females in the earlier part of the 20th century had little power. Swaffield (1988, p.30) suggests that in the nursing and medical professions this resulted in female subordination. She states:

> In caring for the sick, the nurse was to be trained to obey the orders of the doctor in an informed, but subordinate way… It was impossible to develop such a system if there was any higher authority than the male doctor.

This subordination meant that the medical profession was at liberty to develop from a strictly scientific position, which may have led to the demise of the spiritual and religious values once present in nursing. The results of such developments signalled the end of many religious nursing orders. In this sense, health care became less of a vocation, and hospital managers took over the day-to-day control of these institutions.

However, recent announcements signal a possible change in the power relationships within health care – for example, *The NHS Plan: A Plan for Investment, a Plan for Reform* (DH 2000) and, more recently, *The NHS Improvement Plan: Putting People at the Heart of Public Services* (DH 2004). There has also been the introduction of a number of *National Service Frameworks* in an attempt to improve the standards of care for specific client groups. The UK Prime Minister, Tony Blair, has shown concern to reward the expertise of some practitioners by creating new roles within health care such as 'Consultant nurse', or 'Emergency care practitioners'. These possible developments suggest that the medical profession no longer has a monopoly on patient care, that all health care professionals possess expert knowledge and skills and that they can contribute to the ensuing debates concerning health care delivery in the new millennium.

Advances in technology

Activity 1.4

Spend several minutes reflecting upon the technological advancements that have been introduced within health care.

Your reflections may have indicated that health care has witnessed the introduction of numerous technological and clinical advancements specific to your area of practice. For example, within my own discipline, we now have electronic equipment such as digital thermometers, dynamaps for recording vital signs, infusion pumps and care-planning software. We are living in the age of technology. Almost every aspect of patient care can be measured or recorded electronically – the microchip and the computer dominate. It would appear that many tasks once performed by health care professionals are now no longer required (Harrison 1993). One cannot fail to see the advantages that technology has brought to health care and the benefits of such innovations for the health care professional in terms of effectiveness and efficiency in care delivery. However, the greatest hidden danger is that preoccupation with the technological aspects of care may prevent health care professionals from thinking or attending to the spiritual needs of patients. A computer, however effective in measuring blood pressure or central venous pressure, will be unable to communicate the warmth, affection, and sense of care that a single smile can transmit to a patient who may be feeling isolated or alone after admission. The inherent result of a preoccupation with technology is that we fail to see the patient as an individual in the jurisdiction of our care. Burkhardt and Nagai-Jacobson (1994, p.19) share this concern. They write:

> Increasing technology and the multiple pressures of busy clinics and hospitals are among forces that tend to focus efforts on nursing the equipment or treating diagnostic tests. In such times and settings, it is important that nurses remain cognizant of the value of maintaining caring connections with persons undergoing treatments and tests.

Vocation

When tracing the historical heritage of spirituality, the notion of vocation is evident. Individuals in the past entered the nursing and health care professions demonstrating the virtues of selflessness and sacrifice in order to care for those less fortunate. Bradshaw (1996b, p.42) shares this view when she writes: '...for it is clear that throughout history nursing was founded on an ethic and practice of spiritual care embodied in the nurse's vocation.'

It is suggested that today many health care professionals, myself included, may be motivated by economic and capital gain while working in a profession that is saturated in the traditional value of selflessness (Swaffield 1988). Yet one cannot make judgements, because we all need money and security of employment. Indeed, these are often quoted as being fundamental to an individual's spirituality in that they provide meaning, purpose and fulfilment. Therefore, the reasons why individuals enter the nursing and health care professions have changed in that they may not always be altruistic. This may have an indirect effect on the erosion of some of the spiritual values once associated with the notion of vocation. It is quite common now to hear individuals stating that their reason for entering nursing, or possibly any of the health care professions, is to have stability of career or a stepping-stone to a better career. Yet one cannot escape the fact that health care takes a great deal from the individual's emotional and spiritual reserves even if one does not see health care in vocational terms.

Medicalization

One cannot explore the spiritual heritage of health care and its subsequent decline without first examining the notion of medicalization. Some of the points previously discussed are related directly and indirectly to the concept. Medicalization within this section is taken to be a preoccupation with the developments in medical practice at the expense of other aspects of individuals that medicine seeks to serve. McCavery (1985, p.129) draws attention to one of the main dangers associated with medicalization:

> Today, secularization has permeated institutional care and has resulted in the designation of a low priority to all spiritual matters... The result has been an intense interest in the intricacies of medical science and unfortunately, a tendency to accord priority to the disease rather than a person.

As we have previously discussed, within health care the condition that was being treated seemed to be afforded more recognition than the individual that it affected or afflicted. A major concern with medicalization (medical/biological model) is its reductionist or systems-orientated approach, which sees individuals as a disease – for example, a diabetic or an epileptic or schizophrenic. Each of these conditions would be addressed within its own specialty, in the case of diabetes by an endocrinologist, while a neurologist would manage the epilepsy and perhaps a psychiatrist the schizophrenia.

Another concern with medicalization is the misguided view that 'medicine knows best'. If an individual does not conform to expectations – for example, a Jehovah's Witness refuses a blood transfusion – he or she may then be labelled as not conforming and having a disregard for medical opinion that could save his or her life. This point is explored in Case study 1.1.

Medicalization assumes that medicine knows what is best for all individuals who require treatment or are in need of health care. This case study suggests that if the woman had consented to the blood transfusion the outcome might have been different. A positive aspect is that the medical management did abide by the woman's request for no blood – however, retrospectively the feeling was one of loss, sadness and regret – 'if only'. There seems to be a lack of sensitivity here, as individuals are making personal

Case study 1.1 Who knows best?

A young woman is brought into the Accident and Emergency department with a massive gastrointestinal bleed presumed to be oesophageal varices. Immediately the medical and nursing teams start to resuscitate the woman and the consultant asks for four units of blood to be transfused. However, the woman interrupts and states that she does not want the blood transfusion because of her personal beliefs. Therefore, other volume-expanding agents have to be used. Unfortunately, the woman dies from the haemorrhage several hours later. Talk around the department is 'if only the woman had not refused a blood transfusion'. Others say, 'what a waste of life'. Yet the woman's husband says, 'God's will was done and she approached death as she believed was right.'

judgements and allowing their own prejudices towards different religious beliefs to influence their opinions towards the situation. This reaction is not uncommon, as Sampson (1982, p.9) indicates:

> Racial, cultural and religious matters can arouse strong personal feelings and distastes which may have a psychological or physical basis, and the health care community is not immune to them.

Reappraisal of the case study should see individual staff pleased that the woman approached her death with dignity and that she was supported positively in her own personal beliefs and values. This approach seems to be in conflict with medicalization that is concerned at all costs with preserving life and health. It would seem that medicalization and spirituality are incompatible.

The medical model does not look at individuals holistically in that all aspects of a person are interconnected. A physician will look at all the signs and symptoms and the results of investigations to arrive at a diagnosis to treat the system that is diseased or affected. A problem arises when the disease itself is caused by something not physical but psychological, social or spiritual in origin. For example, an elderly lady refuses to eat or drink because she has been taken into residential care and her home sold to pay for her care costs. A nutritional assessment will reveal malnutrition and her urea and electrolytes (U and E) profile will indicate dehydration. The physician may treat both these factors. However, the fundamental issue of her loss of meaning and purpose in life may be neglected if only the medical model is used.

Medicalization of patient care needs to be considered against the individual's own personal beliefs and values. Sampson (1982) highlights a possible solution to the problems linked with medicalization. One suggestion is the development of cultural awareness and cultural sensitivity. The notion that all people working in health care are culturally aware and non-discriminatory is emphasized. This is evident in the vast array of text written on the subject – for example, Henley and Schott (1999), Holland and Hogg (2001) and Sheikh and Gatrad (2000).

Each new medical, surgical or general health care development may have different implications upon a patient's or service user's own personal values or religious beliefs. An example of this may be asking a woman who is having a hysterectomy how she may feel about having to have her ovaries removed and commencing on hormone replacement therapy if this is found to be necessary during the operation. By generating awareness into all aspects of an individual's life, information will be elicited that will enable health care to be provided that will satisfy and take into consideration personal beliefs and values. This approach will go some way to removing the assumption of 'we know what's best' that has been equated with medicalization.

Reversal in opinion

The literature suggests that the spiritual dimension of health care has been eroded and replaced by more secular and modern views. Modernism, secularism and materialism seem to be the guiding forces in health care. Colliton (1981) and Clark *et al.* (1991) indicate that there is a change in opinion, a revitalization and a universal recognition of the importance of refocusing upon patients and service users holistically, paying particular attention to the spiritual dimension. Bradshaw (1994, p.332), commenting upon nursing, writes:

> The lamp has been shattered. To its surprise nursing [I would add health care] finds itself today in the dark, and no matter how it tries to integrate the many different fragments of glass, it cannot achieve the organic unity of care.

Bradshaw highlights the consequences that the erosion of nursing's – indeed health care's – spiritual heritage may have upon caring. Similarly, other professional groups (Culliford 2002; Kirsh *et al.* 2001; Larimore 2001) are advocating a reappraisal of their practice by highlighting the positive role that religion and spirituality may have upon an individual's sense of health and well-being, and suggesting the inclusion of spiritual practice as a way of responding to human diversity (Furman *et al.* 2004). It would appear that health care is now floundering in the dark, seeking direction and a new meaning for its diverse roles and responsibilities.

Activity 1.5

Can you think of any legislation that suggests that health care professionals should be attending to the spiritual needs of their patients?

National

Within the UK, there is an attempt to rediscover and focus upon the spiritual dimension within health care settings which is evident in recent government and political directives. Your reflection may have identified several pieces of national and statutory legislation that currently guide health care practice (Box 1.3). Readers from outside the UK may want to reflect upon their own government's political agenda pertaining to health care, and identify any policies and standards that are relevant to spiritual care.

Box 1.3 Some of the political and professional drivers

Department of Health (1991) *Patient's Charter,* HMSO, London

Department of Health (1992) HSG (92)2: *Meeting the Spiritual Needs of Patients and Staff,* HMSO, London

National Association of Health Authorities and Trusts (1996) *Spiritual Care in the NHS: A Guide for Purchasers and Providers,* National Association of Health Authorities and Trusts, Birmingham

National Council for Hospice and Specialist Palliative Care Services (1997) *Feeling Better: Psychosocial Care in Specialist Palliative Care,* National Council for Hospice and Specialist Palliative Care Services, London

Department of Health (2001) *Your Guide to the NHS,* Department of Health, London

Nursing and Midwifery Council (2002a) *Code of Professional Conduct,* NMC, London

Human Rights Act (1998) www.opsi.gov.uk/acts/acts1998/19980042.htm

Scottish Executive Health Department (2002) *Guidelines on Chaplaincy and Spiritual Care in the NHS in Scotland* (NHS HDL [2002] 76), Scottish Executive, Edinburgh

Department of Health (2003a) *Essence of Care: Patient-focused Benchmarking for Clinical Governance*, Department of Health, London

Department of Health (2003b) *NHS Chaplaincy: Meeting the Religious and Spiritual Needs of Patients and Staff*, Department of Health, London

National Institute for Clinical Excellence (2004) *Improving Supportive and Palliative Care for Adults with Cancer*, National Institute for Clinical Excellence, London

The British government acknowledged the need to focus upon spiritual, cultural and religious issues when they published the Patient's Charter which has now been revised and updated. The Patient's Charter (DH 1991; DH 2001) presents nine Standards. The first Standard deals with issues concerning spirituality: 'NHS staff will respect your privacy and dignity. They will be sensitive to, and respect, your religious, spiritual and cultural needs at all times' (DH 2001, p.29). In the revised version, there is explicit reference to the word 'spiritual'. The inclusion of this word affirms the place that spirituality has within health care, and it signals an attempt by government and policy makers to draw attention to the importance of the spiritual dimension within health care.

Professional

The importance of spirituality has not only been recognized nationally and internationally but also professionally. Readers might want to look at their own governing bodies' regulations and policies to see if reference to the spiritual dimension is evident, for example, in codes of practice. Within my profession, the new governing body for nursing, midwifery and other public health nurses, 'The Nursing and Midwifery Council (NMC)', consulted registrants and other important groups to canvass opinions to update its Code of Professional Conduct (NMC 2004, p.5). The code encourages nurses to address any limitations in their practice knowledge that may be detrimental to their patients' or clients' interests. NMC (2004, p.5) now states:

> You are personally accountable for ensuring that you promote and protect the interests and dignity of patients and clients, irrespective of gender, age, race, ability, sexuality, economic status, lifestyle, culture and religious or political beliefs.

Although there are some changes regarding the content and wording in the new clause, the terms spiritual or spirituality do not feature. Perhaps a possible explanation for this omission is that spirituality permeates and is central to many of the other factors outlined in the clause. Spirituality is shaped by a wide range of factors and forces including culture, and it is individually determined by one's own unique set of beliefs and values. Therefore, if the spiritual dimension is not addressed, then nurses are only partially adhering to the code. One interesting change centres on the tone of language regarding duty of care. There is a shift from recognize in the UKCC (1992) code to you are personally accountable. There is a greater emphasis now placed on the practitioner to meet the litany of needs presented in this clause. The review of your own professional regulatory guidelines may have revealed a similar finding: that spirituality is now perceived as a central component of health care practice.

Statutory

Within many health care professions, as part of registration and quality enhancement, there are now explicit practice competency statements that highlight a specific standard of practice a student must achieve for entry to that particular profession. You may want to look at your own profession and identify if there are any particular competencies that apply to your practice and education. Within my own profession, the NMC (2002b, p.13) in their publication *Requirements for Pre-Registration Nursing Programmes* present the following competency every nursing student ought to achieve for progression into their chosen branch: 'Contribute to the development and documentation of nursing assessments by participating in comprehensive and systematic nursing assessment of the physical, psychological, social and spiritual needs of patients and clients.'

The emphasis of this competency shifts dramatically from participating to undertaking for entry to the register: Undertake and document a comprehensive, systematic and accurate nursing assessment of the physical, psychological, social and spiritual needs of patients, clients and communities. This competency highlights the growing realization by the nursing profession, and again this awareness could be broadened to include all health care professions, that care should be holistic and individualized. This position is a shift or reversal of that which operates around the biological or medical model discussed earlier. The changing climate underlines the responsibility that educational institutions have in providing students involved in all the caring professions with the necessary skills to address and meet patients' spiritual needs in practice. Issues surrounding spirituality and education are explored in greater detail in Chapter 7.

Growing awareness

A search of any of the electronic databases currently available in any university library addressing the subject of spirituality in health care would reveal that since 1990 there has been an explosion of interest in this area. There seems to be a great deal of enthusiasm and passion for this subject with the majority of the health care professions contributing to debate and enquiry. Some of the subjects explored are the language of spirituality, spiritual assessment and issues pertaining to practice and education. This energy and interest that was initially shown by nursing writers in the US has now expanded and the subject is now investigated internationally. This refocusing upon the spiritual dimension which Puchalski and Romer (2000, p.129) term 'non technical aspect of medicine' supports the views presented in this chapter that addressing an individual's spiritual needs may be crucial to that person's health and sense of well-being, something which science and medicine cannot do alone (Thompson 1984).

Within the UK, there has been a proliferation of annual conferences and interest groups addressing the subject of spirituality, and numerous books (at different levels) by different health care professionals have been published. Management's attention has been drawn to the need to assess and evaluate the effectiveness of care provision in this area. To this end, new guidelines (DH 2003b; SEHD 2002) and old and new frameworks (Institute of Nursing 1995; Keighley 1997) for the provision of spiritual care continue to have relevance and importance for the health care professions. This sustained interest and the new initiatives reinforce the attempts by health care theorists, educators and researchers to place the spiritual dimension firmly on the health care agenda, replacing spirituality back at the centre of care delivery. This growing public awareness of the importance of spirituality for an individual's sense of well-being and quality of life has helped to dispel and remove many of the misconceptions that have shrouded spirituality and its place within nursing and the whole of health care (Ross 1995).

The increasing and diverse types of literature and research published on this subject generate new and deeper insights into the spiritual dimension. The growing empirical and conceptual evidence supports the idea that a universal approach and acceptance of the spiritual dimension has emerged challenging all health care professions to evaluate their own attitudes and perceptions towards this fundamental aspect of individualized care. As we move forward in the new millennium it would appear that the technological age is passing, being replaced with recognition of the need to return and reinvest in the caring and spiritual heritage of health care. We are now entering the age of spirituality and spiritual enlightenment. All health care professions and all those involved in the provision of patient and client care need to capitalize and contribute towards this growing debate so that the most efficient and effective care can be developed. Keighley (1997, p.51), in concluding his article addressing the 'Organizational structures and personal spiritual belief' writes:

> Whatever the stimulus, it is clear that there is an opportunity to re-think approaches and structures. If this is achieved in an integrated way, then the benefits to care receivers and caregivers could be very significant indeed.

Conclusion

This chapter traced briefly and superficially some of the historical and modern developments that surround the spiritual heritage of health care. The arguments and evidence presented suggest that the debates concerning the erosion of health care's spiritual heritage and the notion of medicalization are complex and diverse. The emergence of the three 'isms' – modernism, secularism and materialism – indicate that society has lost awareness of things sacred and spiritual. Preoccupation with the technological and material have replaced the notion of holistic and individualized care, at the centre of which rests spirituality. However, it is argued that there is now a reawakening of interest in the spiritual dimension in maintaining an individual's health and sense of well-being. This refocusing upon the spiritual dimension has seen health care, and indeed society, enter a new era of spiritual enlightenment or what Heelas and Woodhead (2005) term 'the spiritual revolution'.

References

Bradshaw, A. (1993) 'Lighting the lamp: the covenant as an encompassing framework for the spiritual dimension of nursing care.' In E. Farmer (ed.) (1996) *Exploring the Spiritual Dimension of Care.* Lancaster: Quay Books.

Bradshaw, A. (1994) *Lighting the Lamp: The Spiritual Dimension of Nursing Care.* London: Scutari Press.

Bradshaw, A. (1996a) 'Does science need religion?' In E. Farmer (ed.) *Exploring the Spiritual Dimension of Care.* Lancaster: Quay Books.

Bradshaw, A. (1996b) 'The legacy of Nightingale.' *Nursing Times 92*, 6, 42–43.

Burkhardt, M.A. and Nagai-Jacobson, M.G. (1994) 'Reawakening spirit in clinical practice.' *Journal of Holistic Nursing 12*, 1, 9–21.

Burnard, P. (1988) 'The spiritual needs of atheists and agnostics.' *Professional Nurse* (December), 130–132.

Carson, V.B. (1989) *Spiritual Dimensions of Nursing Practice.* Philadelphia: WB Saunders.

Clark, C.C., Cross, J.R., Deane, D.M. and Lowry, L.W. (1991) 'Spirituality integral to quality care.' *Holistic Nursing Practice 5*, 3, 67–76.

Cm 5730 (2003) *The Victoria Climbié Inquiry. Report of an Inquiry by Lord Laming.* London: The Stationery Office. Available from www.victoria-climbie-inquiry.org.uk/finreprot/downloadreport.htm

Cobb, M. and Robshaw, V. (eds) (1998) *The Spiritual Challenge of Health Care.* Edinburgh: Churchill Livingstone.

Colliton, M.A. (1981) 'The spiritual dimension of nursing.' In I.L. Beland and J.Y. Passos (eds) *Clinical Nursing*, 4th edn. *New York: Macmillan.*

Cook, C.C.H. (2004) 'Addiction and spirituality.' *Addiction 99*, 539–551.

Culliford, L. (2002) 'Spirituality and clinical care.' *British Medical Journal 325*, 1434–1435.

Cupitt, D. (1997) *After God: The Future of Religion.* London: Weidenfeld and Nicolson.

Dawson, C. (1945) *Progress and Religion: An Historical Enquiry.* London: Sheed and Ward.

Department of Health (DH) (1991) *Patient's Charter.* London: HMSO.

Department of Health (1992) HSG (92)2: *Meeting the Spiritual Needs of Patients and Staff.* London: HMSO.

Department of Health (2000) *The NHS Plan: A Plan for Investment, a Plan for Reform.* London: DH.

Department of Health (2001) *Your Guide to the NHS.* London: Department of Health.

Department of Health (2003a) *Essence of Care: Patient-focused Benchmarking for Clinical Governance.* London: DH.

Department of Health (2003b) *NHS Chaplaincy: Meeting the Religious and Spiritual Needs of Patients and Staff.* London: DH.

Department of Health (2004) *The NHS Improvement Plan: Putting People at the Heart of Public Services.* London: DH.

Donley, R. (1991) 'Spiritual dimensions of health care nursing's mission.' *Nursing and Health Care 12*, 4, 178–183.

Ellis, D. (1980) 'Whatever happened to the spiritual dimension?' *The Canadian Nurse 76*, 8, 42–43.

Furman, L.D., Benson, P.W., Grimwood, C. and Canda, E. (2004) 'Religion and spirituality in social work education and direct practice at the millennium: a survey of UK social workers.' *British Journal of Social Work 34*, 6, 767–792.

Gilliat-Ray, S. (2001) 'Sociological perspectives on the pastoral care of minority faiths in hospital.' In H. Orchard (ed.) (2001) *Spirituality in Health Care Contexts* , 135–146. London: Jessica Kingsley Publishers.

Harrison, J. (1993) 'Spirituality and nursing practice.' *Journal of Clinical Nursing 2*, 211–217.

Heelas, P. and Woodhead, L. (2005) *The Spiritual Revolution.* Oxford: Blackwell Publishing.

Henderson, V. (1966) *Nature of Nursing.* New York: Macmillan.

Henley, A. and Schott, J. (1999) *Culture, Religion and Patient Care in a Multi-Ethnic Society.* London: Age Concern.

Holland, K. and Hogg, C. (2001) *Cultural Awareness in Nursing and Health Care.* London: Arnold.

Human Rights Act (1998) Crown Copyright. Available from: www.opsi.gov.uk/acts/acts1998/19980042.htm Accessed 28/10/05.

Institute of Nursing (1995) *A Framework for Spiritual, Faith and Related Pastoral Care.* Leeds: Institute of Nursing, University of Leeds.

Kearney, S. (1994) 'Spirituality as a coping mechanism in multiple sclerosis: the patient's perspective.' Unpublished BSc dissertation, Hull: Institute of Nursing Studies, University of Hull.

Keighley, T. (1997) 'Organizational structures and personal spiritual belief.' *International Journal of Palliative Nursing 3*, 1, 47–51.

Kirsh, B., Dawson, D., Antolikova, S. and Reynolds, L. (2001) 'Developing awareness of spirituality in occupational therapy students: are our curricula up to the task?' *Occupational Therapy International 8*, 2, 119–125.

Larimore, W.L. (2001) 'Providing basic spiritual care for patients: should it be the exclusive domain of pastoral professionals?' *American Family Physician 63*, 1, 36–40.

Lasagna, L. (1964) *Hippocratic Oath – Modern Version.* Available from: www.pbs.org/wgbh/nova/doctors/oath_modern.html Accessed 30/10/05.

Markham, I. (1998) 'Spirituality and the world faiths.' In M. Cobb and V. Robshaw (eds) (1998) *The Spiritual Challenge of Health Care,* 73–87. Edinburgh: Churchill Livingstone.

McCavery, R. (1985) 'Spiritual care in acute illness.' In P. McGilloway and F. Myco (eds) *Nursing and Spiritual Care.* London: Harper and Row.

Narayanasamy, A. (1997) 'Spiritual dimensions of learning disability.' In B. Gates and C. Beacock (eds) *Dimensions of Learning Disability.* London: Baillière Tindall.

Narayanasamy, A. (1999) 'Transcultural mental health nursing 1: benefits and limitations.' *British Journal of Nursing 8*, 10, 664–668.

Narayanasamy, A. (2001) *Spiritual Care: A Practical Guide for Nurses and Health Care Practitioners,* 2nd edn. Wiltshire: Quay Publishing.

National Association of Health Authorities and Trusts (NAHAT) (1996) *Spiritual Care in the NHS: A Guide for Purchasers and Providers.* Birmingham: NAHAT.

National Council for Hospice and Specialist Palliative Care Services (1997) *Feeling Better: Psychosocial Care in Specialist Palliative Care.* London: National Council for Hospice and Specialist Palliative Care Services.

National Institute for Clinical Excellence (NICE) (2004) *Improving Supportive and Palliative Care for Adults with Cancer.* London: NICE.

Nursing and Midwifery Council (NMC) (2002a) *Code of Professional Conduct.* London: NMC.

Nursing and Midwifery Council (2002b) *Requirements for Pre-Registration Nursing Programmes.* London: NMC.

Nursing and Midwifery Council (2004) *The NMC Code of Professional Conduct: Standards for Conduct, Performance and Ethics.* London: NMC.

Orchard, H. (ed.) (2001) *Spirituality in Health Care Contexts.* London: Jessica Kingsley Publishers.

Orem, D.E. (1985) *Nursing: Concepts of Practice,* 3rd edn. New York: McGraw-Hill.

Peplau, H.E. (1952) *Interpersonal Relations in Nursing.* New York: GP Putnam and Sons.

Puchalski, C. and Romer, A.L. (2000) 'Taking a spiritual history allows clinicians to understand patients more fully.' *Journal of Palliative Medicine 3,* 1, 129–137.

Robbins, C. (1991) 'Spiritual care in a multi-cultural society.' *Pacemaker* (October), 1–3.

Ross, L. (1995) 'The spiritual dimension: its importance to patients' health, well-being and quality of life and its implications for nursing practice.' *International Journal of Nursing Studies 32,* 5, 457–468.

Rumbold, B. (ed.) (2002) *Spirituality and Palliative Care.* Australia: Oxford University Press.

Sampson, C. (1982) *The Neglected Ethic: Religious and Cultural Factors in the Care of Patients.* London: McGraw-Hill.

Scottish Executive Health Department (SEHD) (2002) *Guidelines on Chaplaincy and Spiritual Care in the NHS in Scotland* (NHS HDL [2002] 76). Edinburgh: Scottish Executive.

Sheikh, A. and Gatrad, A.R. (2000) *Caring for Muslim Patients.* Oxon: Radcliffe Medical Press.

Sloan, R.P., Bagiella, E. and Powell, T. (1999) 'Religion, spirituality and medicine.' *The Lancet 353,* 664–667.

Smart, N. (1969) *The Religious Experience of Mankind.* London: Collins.

Swaffield, L. (1988) 'Religious roots.' *Nursing Times 84,* 28–30.

The Shipman Inquiry 2001 Crown Copyright available from: www.the-shipman inquiry.org.uk/home.asp Accessed 10/10/05.

Thompson, J.H. (1984) *Spiritual Considerations in the Prevention, Treatment and Cure of Disease.* London: Oriel Press.

Tournier, P. (1954) *A Doctor's Case Book in the Light of the Bible.* London: SCM Press.

Tournier, P. (1973) *Paul Tournier's Medicine of the Whole Person.* Waco, Texas: Word Books.

Watson, J. (1996) 'Art, caring, spirituality and humanity.' In E. Farmer (ed.) *Exploring the Spiritual Dimension of Care.* Lancaster: Quay Books.

Whipp, M. (1998) 'Spirituality and the scientific mind: a dilemma for doctors.' In M. Cobb and V. Robshaw (eds) (1998) *The Spiritual Challenge of Health Care,* 137–150. Edinburgh: Churchill Livingstone.

Further reading

This selection of literature will develop your understanding and insight into the complex debates surrounding health care's spiritual heritage. These texts will provide a richer and deeper insight into the religious organizations and principles that have shaped and guided health care's spiritual practices.

Bradshaw, A. (1996) 'Does science need religion?' In E. Farmer (ed.) *Exploring the Spiritual Dimension of Care.* Lancaster: Quay Books.

Carson, V.B. (1989) *Spiritual Dimensions of Nursing Practice,* Section 2. Philadelphia: WB Saunders.

Cobb, M. and Robshaw, V. (1998) 'Introduction: body and soul.' In M. Cobb and V. Robshaw (eds) *The Spiritual Challenge of Health Care,* 1–6. Edinburgh: Churchill Livingstone.

Moss, B. (2005) *Religion and Spirituality.* Lyme Regis: Russell House Publishing.

Narayanasamy, A. (1999) 'Learning spiritual dimensions of care from a historical perspective.' *Nurse Education Today 19,* 386–395.

CHAPTER 2

Spirituality Explored

Introduction

This chapter explores the concept of spirituality and explains why it is difficult to define. The chapter demonstrates that spirituality is individually determined and often finds expression and meaning in the ordinary and mundane aspects of life. Definitions of spirituality are presented and discussed within the context of health care. The key terms spiritual need and spiritual well-being, which are used in connection with the spiritual dimension, are introduced.

Making sense

The need to understand and investigate the elusive concept of spirituality has generated much interest and debate within health care. This interest is evident by the abundance of texts now available (Box 2.1).

Box 2.1 A selection of texts written on spirituality

Generic

Cobb and Robshaw (1998)

Farmer (1996)

Orchard (2001)

Robinson, Kendrick and Brown (2003)

Stoter (1995)

Medicine/palliative care/ageing

Aldridge (2000)

Cobb (2001)

Dossey (1993)

Jewell (1998, 2003)

Koenig *et al.* (2001), Koenig (2002)

MacKinlay (2001)

Stanworth (2004)

Sulmasy (1997)

Nursing

Baldacchino (2003)

Bradshaw (1994)

Carson (1989)

Harrison (1993)

McSherry (2000)

Naryanasamy (1991, 2001)

Ross (1997)

Shelly and Fish (1988)

Taylor (2002)

Social/pastoral/mental health

Nash and Stewart (2002)

Rumbold (2002)

Swinton (2001)

Willows and Swinton (2000)

This chapter presents and explores aspects of the spiritual dimension that assist in defining and making sense of the concept in relation to health care. However, a major question arises as to how one can begin to approach and 'make sense' of such diverse, abstract and subjective aspects of holistic health care practice.

Several authors from a range of health care professions (Culliford 2002; Henery 2003; McSherry 2004; Wright 2001, 2002) and from diverse cultures (Rassool 2000; Shirahama and Inoue 2001) have explored and discussed the concept of spirituality. Other commentators have identified an inventory of elements that are perceived as aspects of the spiritual dimension – for example, spiritual needs, spiritual distress, spiritual well-being and a general analysis of the words spirit and spirituality. It would appear that all these terms are interrelated. An investigation into each approach reveals and 'sheds light' on different facets of this multidimensional and mysterious aspect of life.

The lived experience

One way of learning to understand what is meant by the term spirituality is by reflecting upon what the term means to ourselves.

Activity 2.1

Before reading the rest of this chapter, spend a few moments reflecting upon the word spirituality. Write down the thoughts, feelings and images that come to mind while reflecting upon its meaning.

Having undertaken Activity 2.1, you will now appreciate that spirituality is often something that we may not consciously think about and, when asked to describe spirituality, we may find it difficult to articulate either a definition or a description. In describing spirituality, you may have jotted down several points:

- some pertaining to religion such as a belief in a God or a Supreme Being
- more general terms surrounding life such as relationships, beliefs, values, ideologies
- or even issues surrounding death and belief in an after life.

This reflection leads on to Activity 2.2.

Activity 2.2

Having thought about what the word spirituality means to you, now consider and reflect upon the things in life that you most value – e.g. family, friends, health – and anything that is important to you as an individual.

Having thought about the word spirituality and reflected upon the things we value, one starts to appreciate why spirituality is something that we may take for granted. We all have an awareness and sense of importance towards certain things in life (revealed in Activity 2.2) that are personal and unique. By reflecting upon these things, it becomes apparent that everyday rituals, practices and people provide us with much of life's meaning, purpose and fulfilment. However, we may never attach any spiritual significance to them. By spending several moments thinking about the things in life that we value, one can soon produce a list of items – for example, health, family, friends, career, etc. – that are fundamental to our existence and being. An analysis of this list reveals that many of the things that we take for granted link in with the concept of spirituality in that these are aspects of life that generate much of life's meaning, purpose and fulfilment. If we are deprived of any of these because of illness, loss or misfortune, life can soon lose meaning and we can find ourselves questioning our existence at a very deep level, searching for answers and solutions. These important issues will be explored and discussed in a little more depth in the later section, 'The ordinary and mundane'.

Having reflected upon the word spirituality, several important themes begin to emerge. The word spirituality may be interpreted differently by individuals. There is a uniqueness and originality in the way that we perceive the concept. However, what does become evident is that there are certain elements of the subject that are universal and applicable to us all (McSherry and Cash 2004). Spirituality does not only apply to the religious person but to every individual irrespective of religious affiliation. Emerging from this universality is the need for sensitivity when discussing this very personal concept.

Associated terms

To broaden and expand our understanding of the subject of spirituality we need to explore other important aspects and terms that make up the spiritual dimension mentioned earlier in this chapter. Figure 2.1 shows how all the terms associated with spirituality or the spiritual dimension are interrelated and connected. Each term will be addressed in detail throughout the rest of this chapter.

CAUTION

Caution must be used when attempting to define the concept of spirituality, as there is a need for sensitivity. This approach is required because spirituality is a mysterious and complex dimension of our being and existence. It is mysterious in that spirituality involves aspects of daily life that are deeply personal and sensitive, such as religion and religious affiliation, and it is complex in that it involves aspects of life that are intimately interwoven into the tapestry of beliefs, values and cultures. These are all aspects of life that individuals may find hard to discuss, define and talk about openly (think back to Activity 2.1 – did you find it difficult?). In conclusion, the individual interprets spirituality differently. This interpretation will be influenced by personal identity and life experiences. This must be borne in mind when trying to define spirituality because there is always the danger of applying our own definitions of spirituality to others. This can only be avoided if we are sensitive and understand the personal nature of spirituality in a non-judgemental way.

The human spirit defined

Origins of the word

The word 'spirit' has its origins from the Latin word 'spiritus', which generates images of life, breath, wind and air. The word 'spirit' relates to the unique spirit of an individual that is their life force, the essence and energy of their being. It is this force that develops in an individual the ability to transcend the natural laws and orders of this life, allowing access to a mysterious or transcendent dimension. The 'spirit' drives and motivates individuals to find meaning and purpose, allowing expression in all aspects and experiences of life, especially in times of crisis and need.

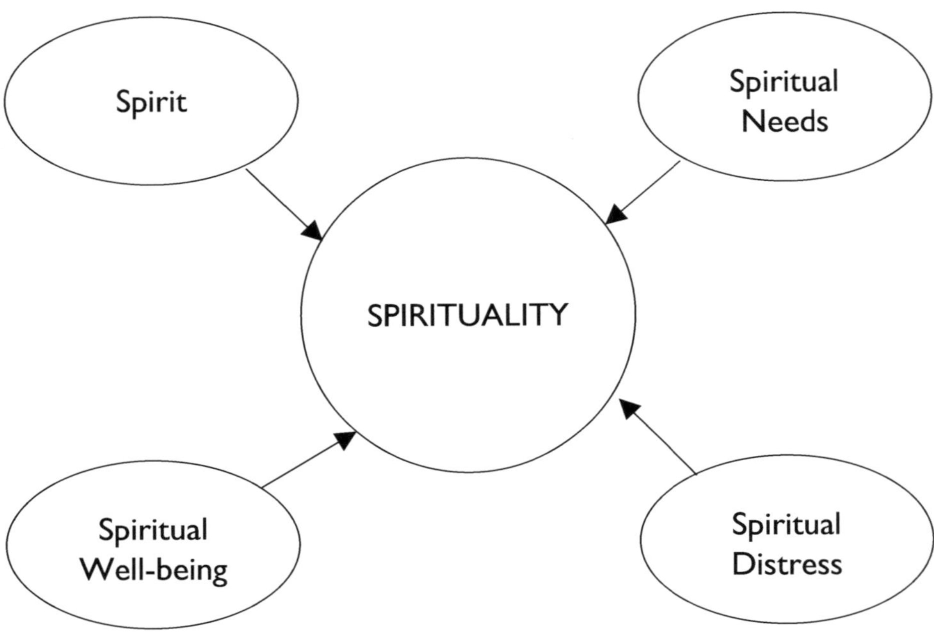

Figure 2.1: Terms associated with spirituality

Meanings associated with the word

Several authors (Coyle 2002; Dickinson 1975; Shelly and Fish 1988; Stoll 1989; Tanyi 2002) have investigated the concept of spirituality by first exploring possible meanings associated with the word 'spirit'. Everyday usage of the word is illustrated by the definition in *The New Oxford Dictionary of English*, which provides two descriptions of the word that may help to demystify its use within health care:

> 1. of, relating to, or affecting the human spirit or soul as opposed to material or physical things...
> 2. of, relating to, religion or religious belief.
>
> (Pearsall 1998, p.1794)

The above definitions suggest that the 'spirit' of a person is an entity on its own. They also suggest that it is an animating life force present within all individuals. It is also described as a frame of mind or attitude towards life.

Stoll (1989) describes a person's spirit as the *Imago dei* (Image of God) that is present within every person, making him or her a thinking, feeling, moral, creative being able to relate meaningfully to God (as defined by the person), self and others. Stoll is referring directly to the *Book of Genesis* (2: 7), which reads: 'Yahweh God fashioned man of dust from the soil. Then he breathed into his nostrils a breath of life, and thus man became a living being.' This quotation infers that it is this 'breath of life' that distinguishes and separates humankind from the rest of the animal kingdom because individuals are made in the likeness of God, whose presence resides within them in a mystical union. This perspective is orientated and focused in the Judeo-Christian tradition. Yet even the atheist and agnostic still possess a spirit or attitude towards life (Burnard 1988). The suggestion of an animating force or principle is supported by Dickinson (1975, p.1790), who states: 'Spirit is the animating but intangible principle that gives liveliness to the physical organism as well as the literal breath of life.'

Definitions of spirituality

After exploring the word 'spirit', the next step is to try and define what is meant by the word 'spirituality'. It was stated earlier that the concept of spirituality is gaining much attention within the health care literature. A study of some of these articles and texts soon reveals that some of the definitions presented are very descriptive, anecdotal and rhetorical, presenting the views and opinions of individuals, which cannot be generalized and applied to the general population (Bradshaw 1996; MacLaren 2004; McSherry 1996; Turner 1996; Wright 1997). However, these publications do contribute to our understanding of the concept in that they provide us with an insight into what people feel and think about spirituality.

Among the numerous descriptive definitions of spirituality that are to be found in the literature, there are several that have been developed and used in research studies to provide a framework for investigation. One such definition of spirituality, which has been quoted and referred to in many texts, is that presented by Murray and Zentner (1989, p.259). According to these authors, spirituality is:

> A quality that goes beyond religious affiliation, that strives for inspirations, reverence, awe, meaning and purpose, even in those who do not believe in any good. The spiritual dimension tries to be in harmony with the universe, and strives for answers about the infinite, and comes into focus when the person faces emotional stress, physical illness or death.

If we read this definition several times and reflect upon its meaning and significance to health care, several important themes may begin to emerge:

- spirituality is a universal concept relevant to all individuals
- the uniqueness of each individual is paramount
- formal religious affiliation is not a prerequisite of spirituality
- an individual may become more spiritually aware during a time of need.

This definition highlights the complex and subjective nature of spirituality, reinforcing the notion of mystery and transcendence. It demonstrates how all aspects of life – physical, psychological and social – are interrelated and interconnected. From this definition it would appear that spirituality is concerned with an individual's past, present and future, especially when facing illness or the prospect of death. Reed (1992, p.350) adopts a similar description of spirituality when she writes:

> Specifically spirituality refers to the propensity to make meaning through a sense of relatedness to dimensions that transcend the self in such a way that empowers and does not devalue the individual. This relatedness may be experienced intrapersonally (as a connectedness within oneself), interpersonally (in the context of others and the natural environment) and transpersonally (referring to a sense of relatedness to the unseen, God, or power greater than the self and ordinary source).

Reed's definition suggests that spirituality is concerned with the individual and his or her relationship with others and the environment, also reaffirming the notion that spirituality involves an awareness of something greater or beyond oneself (the mystical nature inherent in every individual).

Earlier you were asked (Activity 2.2) to reflect upon the things in life that bring you value and meaning. The two definitions of spirituality presented in this chapter suggest that it embraces all aspects of life that bring value and meaning, since they imply that spirituality is concerned with everyday events and concerns such as relationships, health, career, etc. Academics may argue that this is an oversimplification of the concept. However, if spirituality is to be relevant to health care and applied in clinical practice, then spirituality must be defined in a manner that makes it both meaningful and relevant for patients and all working within health care. A noticeable omission in the literature (particularly nursing) is that many definitions of spirituality have been constructed and perpetuated without any real criticality or analysis of them in terms of relevance to individuals and practice. Taylor (2002) and McSherry and Cash (2004) present tables in chronological order to show how spirituality has been defined within nursing and health care.

The ordinary and mundane

During a workshop on spirituality, one of the co-facilitators, a chaplain, made a useful observation concerning the word 'spirituality'. Incorporated in the middle of the word 'spirituality' is found the word 'ritual', a word well known by nurses (Walsh and Ford 1989) and all health care professionals. What has this point to do with spirituality? Ritual means a regulated or repeated action, and this can be applied to religious practices and ordinary aspects of life. Within the context of a religious ceremony prayers or actions are carried out according to historical customs and practices – for example, the marriage ceremony. An example from nursing may be the ritual of recording daily observations without really asking if they are necessary. It would appear that all individuals require ritual and routine because they provide structure and security. Therefore, if one applies these principles to spirituality, it would seem that the word is concerned with ordinary events and routines of daily living. The definition offered by Murray and Zentner supports the idea that spirituality is concerned with the ordinary and mundane ritualistic events of life. This may appear a contradiction since the use of the word 'mundane' implies an absence of the spiritual. However, if one reflects upon daily living, it is often the mundane rituals such as going to work, doing the washing or walking the dog that bring meaning and purpose to everyday life. As suggested earlier, these ordinary and often mundane tasks are usually taken for granted, and the fulfilment derived from them is not recognized until an event occurs that causes a break in normal practices.

This is illustrated in Case study 2.1. John's situation highlights that it is the everyday tasks and rituals that give structure, meaning and purpose. Nurses will encounter numerous patients like John who are trying to find new meaning as their roles and lives change. It is important to recognize that spirituality is not just concerned with matters of theology and existential beliefs, but about the ordinary and the mundane.

One important point to consider when trying to establish a definition of spirituality is not to make the subject complex and produce a definition that may be authoritative. The way forward is to think of spirituality in terms of its relevance and importance to individuals in their everyday existence. All people irrespective of creed, culture, race or religion have a spirituality that is uniquely interpreted and determined by their everyday situation.

Case study 2.1 Finding meaning in the ordinary and mundane

John, aged 75, is admitted into hospital with a chest infection. While admitting John, the nurse enquires about his occupation. He replies, 'I'm recently retired. I was a school teacher – and do you know something? I didn't think I'd miss it – all the hassle – when I retired, but I do! Life seems to have lost some of its meaning, now that I don't work.'

Spirituality does not only equal religion

In an article entitled 'The inner light', Allen (1991) suggests that nurses would be more scandalized to find a Bible in a patient's property bag than a copy of the *Karma Sutra*. Allen is highlighting the misconceptions surrounding spirituality and religion. In the past, the word spirituality has been used synonymously with religion. Any mention of the word spirituality either implied that a patient required the services of the hospital chaplain or that a nurse who attended to such patients was in need of a psychiatric referral. If one adopts such a narrow definition of the word and applies it only to the religious and pious, then there is a danger that a large proportion of patients and indeed nurses may not have their spiritual needs addressed. For some individuals, patients, service users and health care professionals, the religious aspect and the belief in a God will be fundamental and central to their interpretation of spirituality. However, if this definition were applied to all individuals, it would be extremely inappropriate and possibly offensive. It appears that in today's society these two words are in conflict or opposition – the spiritual/religious versus the secular and materialistic. Yet this conflict only arises if one chooses to be judgemental in the interpretation of the word spirituality by adopting a narrow definition. Tolerance, understanding and flexibility have to be used and applied when defining spirituality. Only by being tolerant to each individual's religious orientation or political and philosophical persuasion will a true understanding of spirituality be gained. If one adopts this approach, then these two words will not be viewed in opposition but as elements or threads that contribute and make up the larger tapestry of spirituality.

Analogy and symbolism

The word spirituality is perceived and used differently by all individuals. By adopting this individualist approach, the meaning of the word becomes mysterious and subjective in that the term may mean different things to individuals within differing contexts. One way in which individuals, and indeed societies, try to describe or define the word is by using analogy and symbolism. An example can be found in the way that religions use drawings to illustrate their God(s). Ancient peoples drew figures of animals that they worshipped because they provided food. This approach can be applied to spirituality because images or illustrations with which people are familiar assist in providing visual stimulation and insight, allowing the hidden meanings or interpretations of the word to be revealed.

MOUNTAIN RANGE

Life is depicted as a journey or pilgrimage. Sometimes the route and the scenes are beautiful and idyllic. Yet there are times when the mountains are steep and difficult to ascend, and no sooner does one conquer one peak than another appears on the horizon that is much higher and steeper. Life and spirituality is like this for most individuals. At one period in time a person may be experiencing hardship and conflict that may be manifested as illness, disease or bereavement (the steep slopes). Yet there are many occasions when a person experiences joy and happiness, life is running smoothly and calmly, and everything seems to fall into place with little effort (the scenic routes). This analogy suggests that life can be difficult and that at some point events may occur that confront, challenge and test us. It is during this journey that a person's spirituality is shaped and developed. This raises the notion that spirituality can be developed. In fact several authors have suggested that spirituality changes and evolves across a lifespan (Carson 1989; Erikson 1963). Our spirituality is not completed overnight, nor is it something static; rather it is transient and always in a state of flux. It is the spirit's ability to adjust and change to situations, either religious or secular, that will ultimately shape an individual's spirituality.

A FOOTBALL

The world cup and league football provide entertainment for many, and hopefully joy for the victorious. The football (Fig. 2.2) provides another analogy for spirituality (McSherry and Draper 1998). Here we consider that spirituality is made up of many component parts (patches) all stitched together to

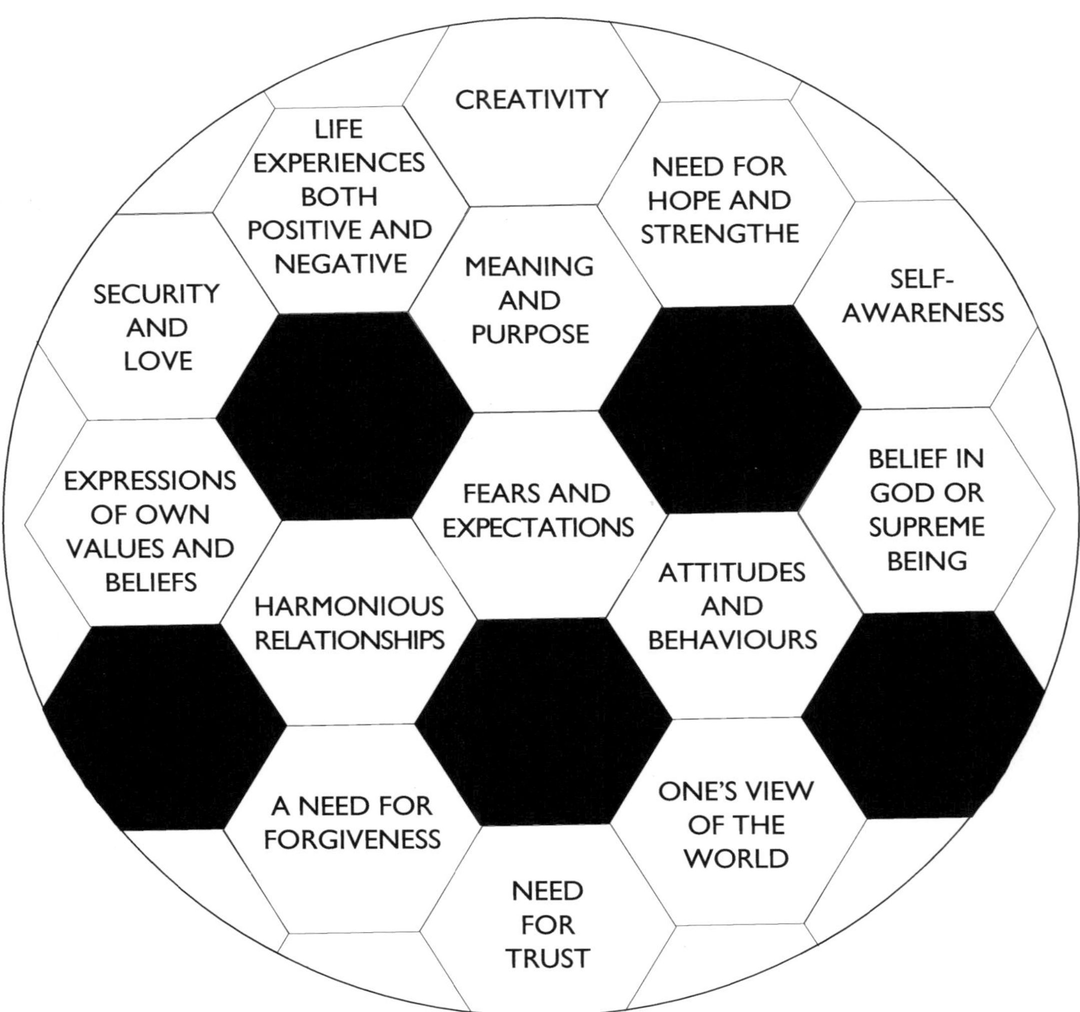

Figure 2.2: The analogy of spirituality as a football shows the complexity of the concept involving many dimensions

make the person (ball) . The synthetic patches each represent a different aspect of spirituality. Each aspect is attached and interrelated to the next because they are stitched tightly together. All the patches share the same importance and cannot function in isolation. The football can be burst and/or punctured, requiring repair. This happens in both daily life and the spiritual life, when occasionally circumstances occur that knock the air out of us. These events are usually unexpected and beyond our control. Often the person is left asking the question 'why?', and searching for some meaning or purpose in the event. The football takes many kicks during the match – here the match represents the arena of life and the ball represents our spirituality or the individual.

Spiritual needs

As living functional, volitional and interactive creatures we have certain basic physiological, social and psychological needs that are fundamental to our survival – for example, a physical need for food and water (Dunn 1993). Deprived of these necessities for prolonged periods, we soon dehydrate, starve and die.

Labun (1988) suggests that spirituality is expressed and shaped by the accepted practices and beliefs of a particular culture. This approach to spirituality implies that spiritual needs have their origin in the institutional religious domains, intimating a belief in God or a deity. It appears that spiritual needs have an intrinsic and extrinsic value and meaning: their relevance and value to the individual is intrinsic, and their relationship with the universe at large is extrinsic. Stallwood and Stoll (1975, p.1088) define spiritual needs as:

> Any factors necessary to establish and maintain a person's dynamic personal relationship with God (as defined by that individual)...and out of that relationship to experience forgiveness..., love..., hope..., trust...meaning and purpose in life.

Activity 2.3

There exists within nursing a debate surrounding spiritual needs. What are they, and do we all have spiritual needs?

Stallwood and Stoll demonstrate that spiritual needs are not purely associated with religion or belief in God but a semantic philosophy towards life (a search for meaning and purpose). Colliton (1981) stresses that spiritual needs are a requirement that touches the core of one's being where the search for personal meaning takes place.

Victor Frankl (1987, p.74), a survivor of the World War II concentration (extermination) camps and the founder of a Vienna School of Existential Psychotherapy, stresses people's search for meaning and purpose when he states:

> The prisoner who had lost faith in the future – his future – was doomed. With his loss of belief in the future, he also lost his spiritual hold; he let himself decline and become subject to mental and physical decay.

Frankl goes on to say that meaning must be specific and have purpose to the individual. Travelbee (1966, p.vii) believes that:

> A major belief is that human beings are motivated by a search for meaning in all life experiences, and meaning can be found in the experiences of illness, suffering and pain.

It is the health care professionals' role to assist individuals to make sense and find meaning in such times of crisis such as the acceptance of a terminal diagnosis, the loss of a loved one, or adapting to life with a permanent disability. These approaches presented by Frankl (1987) and Travelbee (1966) suggest that spiritual needs are seen as the deepest requirements of self. If an individual is able to identify and fulfil these requirements, then he or she can function harmoniously, finding meaning, value, purpose and hope in life even when life may be threatened (Harrison 1993).

Several authors (Highfield and Cason 1983; Narayanasamy 1991, 2001; Shelly and Fish 1988; Taylor 2002) have identified and categorized a litany of items that can be included in the classification of spiritual needs. Shelly and Fish (1988) identified three spiritual needs:

- the need for meaning and purpose
- the need for love and relatedness
- the need for forgiveness.

It must be stressed that Shelly and Fish base their work upon a Judeo-Christian approach to spirituality. Therefore, for the Christian it is Jesus Christ who is identified as the main person able to satisfy all people's deepest yearnings and spiritual needs. Shelly and Fish suggest that nurses – indeed all health care professionals – may be called upon to function in a pastoral role, in order that a patient's spiritual and religious needs are addressed during periods of hospitalization, social deprivation or he or she is isolated or prevented from maintaining his or her own unique individual religious practices.

Highfield and Cason (1983) used a spiritual needs approach in their descriptive study investigating surgical nurses' awareness of spiritual concerns. The researchers identified four spiritual needs:

- the need for meaning and purpose in life
- the need to give and receive love
- the need for hope
- the need for creativity.

Interestingly, Highfield and Cason leave the definition or interpretation of God up to the individual's own perceptions and beliefs. The work of these authors broadens and widens the boundaries of spiritual needs. There is a shift away from the religious aspects of life to include other fundamental and valuable concepts – which are still spiritual in origin – although the main thrust focuses around meaning and purpose, fulfilment and value in life.

Narayanasamy (1991, 2001) highlights the inclusion of other spiritual needs by applying the concept directly to nursing and latterly to health care. Like the previous authors, he lists:

- the need for meaning and purpose
- the need for love and harmonious relationships
- the need for forgiveness
- the need for a source of hope and strength
- creativity.

However, he identifies and lists a further four spiritual needs:

- the need for trust
- the need for expression of personal beliefs and values
- the need for spiritual practices
- expressions of God or deity.

These spiritual needs are explained in more detail in Box 2.2. They demonstrate that a spiritual need may originate from any facet of our human existence, whether it be physiological, psychological or sociological. It stresses the importance of an holistic approach to health care. There is a dynamic interplay and exchange of the spiritual dimension with all the other realms of our existence. The confusion arises when a spiritual need is viewed in isolation or when an individual is fragmentalized, thus obscuring the whole meaning. An individual may express a need for a harmonious relationship, after having experienced a marital breakdown. The more psychologically oriented may see this as a psychological need, when in reality the individual is expressing a desire to explore issues that are fundamental, unique and central to their existence – spiritual in nature, originating from the psychosocial dimensions. Likewise, it would be a grave misconception and error to infer that an atheist or an agnostic does not have spiritual needs because they do not share a belief in a God or deity (Burnard 1988).

Assessing spiritual needs

Bradshaw (1972) produced a taxonomy of social need distinguishing and stressing the interaction between normative, felt, expressed and comparative need. Cobb (1998) tells us this type of needs classification has been used in

Box 2.2 Spiritual needs explained

Meaning and purpose

We all have a desire and need to identify some meaning in our lives and existence that will assist in generating motivation or purpose, which will lead to a sense of fulfilment. This search is undertaken in health and during times of illness.

Love and harmonious relationships

Without the intimacy and comfort gained by sharing with others – e.g. a spouse, partner or close friends – we can feel isolated, alone and deprived of touch, security and love. These are all important needs derived from personal contact and involvement with people. However, can the same love be generated or experienced by close contact with animals and creation? An observation has been made by several students that relationships are not always harmonious and that individuals can grow and learn from all experiences.

Need for forgiveness

At times life can be troublesome and conflicts do emerge. However, unresolved anger and guilt can lead to loss of physical, psychological, social and spiritual well-being. Therefore, in order to maintain an equilibrium, there is a need to try and resolve conflict in life and at times forgiveness is sought.

Need for a source of hope and strength

Spirituality is often referred to as a source of inner strength and hope. Personal beliefs, values and attitudes can bring hope in people, the future or from a religious perspective, such as life everlasting, enabling individuals to draw strength from their convictions and commitment.

Creativity

The ability to find meaning, expression and value in aspects of life such as literature, art, music and other activities, which originate from the creative nature of individuals, provides expression and meaning as well as a means of communication. Creativity can be inspirational, elevating people's emotions and feelings to the beauty present in creation.

Trust

Individuals can become isolated and neglected when deprived of trust. Trust can be applied to the individual, family, friends or society – the world at large. Trust is a prerequisite for establishing friendships and therapeutic relationships. By adopting this approach, it would appear that trust is fundamental to existence and communication. Trust leads to a sense of value, self-worth and acceptance by others.

Ability to express one's own personal beliefs and values

In life there is a fundamental need to express one's own personal beliefs and values. This need is fostered in many modern societies. The inability to express one's own personal beliefs and values can lead to frustration and eventually hostility.

Maintain spiritual practices

As we progress through life, certain spiritual practices may be developed and fashioned. These practices may originate from within a religious framework, such as the need for daily prayer or attendance at church services or the synagogue, mosque or temple. However, an individual may have grown spiritually through a weekly walk in the countryside or by taking part in sports. During periods of illness or hospitalization, there will be a need to ensure such practices are continued where possible.

Express one's own belief in God or deity

An important dimension of spirituality for some individuals is the belief in a God or supreme power or being. This may be a belief in a God who is creator of the world (Judeo-Christian tradition). However, for some individuals their supreme being or deity may be their work or recreational activity. A flexible approach is required since God or deity is defined by the individual.

undertaking the health needs assessments that are used in the strategic planning of health services. Similarly, within my own profession, the concept of need has been debated in nursing models with some now stressing the importance of spiritual needs ('the spiritual variable' described in *The Neuman Systems Model* (Neuman 1995) and other nursing and health care models will be discussed in Chapter 3). Case study 2.2 provides an example of a situation where a patient has spiritual needs.

Case study 2.2 Time to think

Jim, 65 years old, was admitted to the ward with a grossly swollen right leg, thigh and calf. A diagnosis of DVT (deep vein thrombosis) was made. He was started on a heparin infusion and kept on total bed rest because of the severe pain when he mobilized.

One morning while the nurse was talking to Jim he became very emotional and began to cry. As the nurse listened to him, it emerged that on 24 December it was the first anniversary of his wife's death. Jim recalled how he had been married for 45 years and for the last 10 years of his married life had been the main carer for his wife, who suffered from rheumatoid arthritis. Jim went on to describe how lonely and depressed he felt, stating that a day did not pass without him thinking about his wife and the wonderful life they had shared together. Jim was not a religious man but he did believe in life after death. Could you identify Jim's spiritual needs?

After reading this case study you probably identified several spiritual needs that Jim was experiencing:

- loss of meaning, purpose and fulfilment
- the death of his wife and the loss of a very long loving relationship
- Jim has lost hope and motivation in his own abilities and the future
- there is a need for trust so that Jim can discuss his anxieties and needs in a secure and confidential environment.

Reading this case study illustrates how spiritual needs may present themselves and how they are often interrelated. Jim appears to have lost the ability to find meaning, purpose and fulfilment in his life. The anniversary of his wife's death is approaching and memories and emotions are evoked that remind him that a fundamental part of his life – the relationship and love experienced with his wife – has 'ended'. Jim finds himself alone, isolated and depressed. We may well argue that what Jim is experiencing is a natural grieving process, and correctly so, but Jim is also questioning his life at a very deep level, trying to establish some order and sense so that he can move forward to regain stability. (These issues will be discussed later in Chapter 4.)

When addressing spiritual needs, there is a need for sensitivity, self-awareness and personal value clarification (we must know ourselves) (Harrison and Burnard 1993). Some individuals' spiritual needs may arise and be developed within a religious framework, as they have a substantive belief in a God or deity and follow the teachings and ideologies of that particular religion. Yet others may find meaning, purpose and value in life by investing energy in relationships, work, hobbies, etc. There are no restrictions or constraints dictating what constitutes a spiritual need. A spiritual need is unique, specifically determined and interpreted or perceived by the individual who demonstrates or expresses that need.

Spiritual distress

If we all have a spirituality and spiritual needs, then logically it must follow that when a crisis or sudden event occurs in life we may experience not only physical, psychological and social distress but also spiritual distress. Burnard (1987, p.377) states that: 'Spiritual distress is the result of total inability to invest life with meaning. It can be demotivating, painful and can cause anguish to the sufferer.' This definition or approach implies loss of function, dispiritedness and a recognition of behaviour or feelings that convey an altered spiritual integrity. Labun (1988) has identified seven human experiences that demonstrate an altered spiritual integrity, or spiritual distress: spiritual pain, alienation, anxiety, guilt, anger, loss and despair. These demotivating and debilitating experiences and behaviour suggest that the person becomes dysfunctional, withdrawn and unable to invest or relate to life in a meaningful and integrating manner. There is a disturbance in the flow of energy from the spiritual dimension to the other dimensions. This loss of equilibrium or disturbance may be the result of several aetiological or contributing factors, some pathophysiological and some situational in origin – for example, disease, illness, marital or relationship breakdown, loss/bereavement (think back to Case study 2.2). Not all patients or service users will present with spiritual needs, despite experiencing illness or some crisis in their life. This finding was certainly evident in my research (McSherry 2004).

If one approaches spiritual development across the lifespan, then there are stages within our human development that are often troublesome and confusing – for example, adolescence or old age – when one is forced to ask questions and establish meaning (Carson 1989; MacKinlay 2001; Smith and McSherry 2004). These periods of questioning and uncertainty in life can result in spiritual distress. If an individual is unable to find meaning in life or the experience causes spiritual pain, spiritual distress, dispiritedness and spiritual collapse, the result may be that the individual experiences inner turmoil, conflict and confusion. There is a need to confer order and find meaning in the situation that has caused the disharmony and distress. From a religious and mystical perspective, this period of search and confusion has been called the 'dark night of the soul' described vividly by the Carmelite mystic, St John of the Cross.

This classification or category of human experiences has been tentatively recognized as a nursing diagnosis by The National Group for Classification of Nursing Diagnosis. Carpenito (2000, p.451), in the book *Nursing Diagnosis: Application to Clinical Practice*, describes spiritual distress as: 'The state in which the individual or group experiences or is at risk of experiencing a disturbance in the belief or value system that provides strength, hope, and meaning to life.'

Signs of spiritual distress

The defining characteristics focus primarily upon a disturbance in the individual's belief and value system, which may manifest itself in uncertainty, ambivalence and a sense of emptiness or aloneness. The individual may display other traits such as:

- anger
- fear
- a morbid preoccupation with suffering and death.

As individuals, we all search and have a desire to establish order in our lives by discovering meaning and purpose. The challenge of the health care professions is to assist individuals who are spiritually distressed, dispirited, and at times emotionally and physically dysfunctional, to explore life's crisis in an attempt to rediscover meaning and value so that once again they can invest positively in life.

Spiritual well-being

A logical argument exists in that if we can experience spiritual distress then we must at times experience a sense of spiritual well-being. Hungelmann *et al.*

(1985, p.152) describe spiritual well-being as a state of acceptance of self/others and a positive disposition towards life when they write:

> ...a sense of harmonious interconnectedness between self, others/nature, and ultimate other which exists throughout and beyond time and space. It is achieved through a dynamic and integrative growth process which leads to realization of the ultimate purpose and meaning of life.

This description implies that in order to experience spiritual well-being an individual must achieve harmonious interconnectedness, peace and acceptance within all dimensions of his or her existence and being as he or she progresses through the different developmental stages and experiences of life. It requires an individual to be introspective and reflective, thus revealing the meaning and the purpose so that consolidation and ultimate acceptance can occur.

Hungelmann *et al.* demonstrate that there is a definite change of focus from the religious (theistic) approaches to spiritual well-being as presented by Byrne, who refers to the definition given by the White House Conference on Aging (cited in Byrne 1985) – 'the affirmation of life in a relationship with God, self, community and environment which nurtures and celebrates wholeness.' – to a realization of a further dimension that has socio-psychological components (Harrison 1993). The definition implies that there are two distinct, interactive dimensions to spiritual well-being. There is a transcendental or existential relationship with an ultimate other and a purely physio-psychosocial relationship involving the individual with their environment/world and other individuals. These dimensions have been identified by the sociologist Morberg (1971, 1979) and nurse theorist Stoll (1989). They suggest that there is a vertical dimension, referring to the individual's sense of well-being in relation to their God, and a horizontal dimension, referring to the person's sense of life purpose or satisfaction with their state in the world (Figure 2.3). This two-dimensional, dualist approach is very similar to the 'conceptual model of the nature of man' developed by Stallwood and Stoll (1975) (discussed in Chapter 3). These approaches to spiritual well-being demonstrate that conceptualization and definition will be difficult because of the numerous factors and variables involved. Nevertheless, this approach emphasizes the interactive and integrative nature of both the vertical and horizontal dimensions, which cannot be viewed in isolation.

Emerging debates

In an attempt to sharpen our understanding, Ellison (1983) proposes that spiritual well-being may not be the same thing as spiritual health. The debate emerging is – are they not the one and same thing? Ellison (1983, p.332) states: 'If we are spiritually healthy we will feel generally alive purposeful, and fulfilled, but only to the extent that we are psychologically healthy as well.' This statement stresses the intimate relationship that spiritual well-being has with the psychological dimension. Yet there exists a danger of misinterpretation since this statement infers that spiritual well-being is determined by our psychological state. It fails to accept spiritual well-being or spirituality as a separate entity, which unifies and integrates in a mystical manner all dimensions of our being. Byrne (1985, p.32) subscribes to this philosophy when she states: 'Emotional support alone will not suffice if the person's problem is spiritual in nature.'

Byrne seems to distinguish the spiritual from the emotional and the psychological realms. Reed (1987, p.336) writes: 'spiritual transcendence does not imply a detachment from other dimensions of one's life,' thus emphasizing the unifying and permeating nature of spirituality. Neuman (1995, p.29) shares this approach when describing the spiritual variable incorporated in her nursing model:

> The author views it as being on a continuum of development that permeates all other client system variables. The client/client system can move from complete unawareness of this variable's presence and potential, or even denial of it, to a consciously and highly developed spiritual understanding that supports client optimal wellness; that is, the spirit controls the mind, and the mind consciously or unconsciously controls the body...

Leggieri (1986, p.50) refers to the integrating approach to spiritual well-being, stating: 'Therefore healing must take place on all levels of life because the separate forces work together as an integrated whole within persons.'

Spiritual well-being (spiritual health) will be determined by both vertical and horizontal dimensions functioning harmoniously and dynamically together, fostering a positive and meaningful attitude and disposition towards life. Figure 2.3 underlines this dynamic relationship between the person and their relationship with the horizontal and vertical dimensions. In order to have spiritual well-being, a person would feel integrated, finding meaning and purpose within both the vertical and the horizontal dimensions. These two dimensions do not function in isolation since to adopt such an approach

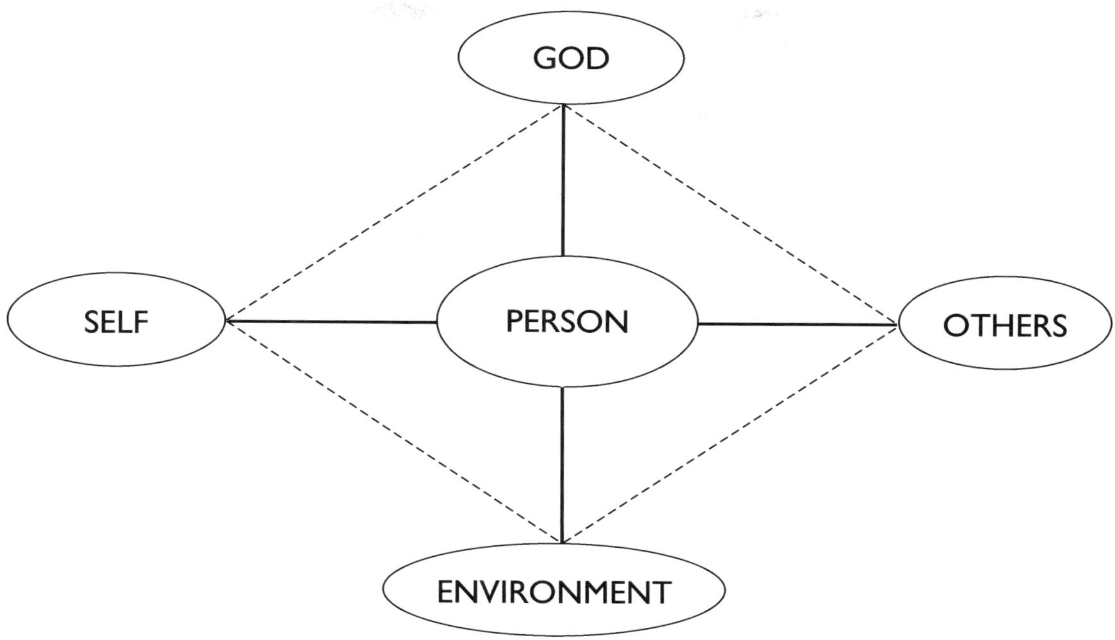

Figure 2.3: The relationship between the horizontal and vertical dimensions of spirituality (adapted from Stoll 1989)

would be reductionist, suggesting that spirituality is detached from the physical world. These arguments will be further explored in Chapter 3.

By adopting this approach, there exists a danger of reducing spiritual well-being to a purely functional, observable and measurable level. If spirituality is transcendent and existential (we have a say in our own destiny), then how can it be reduced to a functional state? Stoll (1989, p.19) states: 'Spiritual well-being is not a state but rather is indicative of the presence of spiritual health in the person.' Therefore, spiritual well-being is identified as behavioural expressions of spiritual health.

As a result, spiritual well-being is not just a functional state but the expression of an underlying state that is the essence and core of one's being. Ellison (1983, p.332) writes:

> If this is an accurate conception we are freed from the burden of trying to exactly or empirically measure the inner contours of one's spirit – a task which is most likely impossible.

All these approaches to the concept of spiritual well-being highlight that there is a need for further clarification, categorization and refinement of the term. There is now emerging a great deal of debate on what constitutes spirituality, but Morrison's (1989) concerns that conceptual writings (and I would add analytical) on the subject of spiritual well-being remain sparse is still relevant. Ensuing debate on the spiritual dimension will ensure clarity and a degree of commonality in definition instead of confusion and possible distortion.

Activity 2.4

Having briefly explored the concept of spiritual need, spend a little time reflecting upon your own life and identify any spiritual needs that are important to you.

Conclusion

This chapter has explored possible definitions associated with the word 'spirituality'. It has asked you to reflect upon your own understanding of the word in order to clarify meaning and understanding in respect of daily living. Terms associated with spirituality have been discussed and where possible related to health care practice. The complex and subjective nature of spirituality was revealed and it is suggested that creating an authoritative definition may be difficult. The definitions and arguments developed indicate that spirituality can be applied to all things secular, temporal and mystical. However, there are still many questions that need to be answered if spirituality is to be fully understood and defined.

References

Aldridge, D. (2000) *Spirituality, Healing and Medicine Return to the Silence.* London: Jessica Kingsley Publishers.

Allen, C. (1991) 'The inner light.' *Nursing Standard 5*, 20, 52–53.

Baldacchino, D. (2003) *Spirituality in Illness and Care.* Malta: Perca Library.

Bradshaw, A. (1994) *Lighting the Lamp: The Spiritual Dimension of Nursing Care.* London: Scutari Press.

Bradshaw, A. (1996) 'The legacy of Nightingale.' *Nursing Times 92*, 6, 42–43.

Bradshaw, J.R. (1972) 'A taxonomy of social need.' In G. McLachlan (ed.) *Problems and Progress in Medical Care*, 69–82. Oxford: Oxford University Press.

Burnard, P. (1987) 'Spiritual distress and the nursing response: theoretical considerations and counselling skills.' *Journal of Advanced Nursing 12*, 377–382.

Burnard, P. (1988) 'The spiritual needs of atheists and agnostics.' *Professional Nurse 4*, 3, 130–132.

Byrne, M. (1985) 'A zest for life!' *Journal of Gerontological Nursing 11*, 4, 30–33.

Carpenito, L.J. (2000) *Nursing Diagnosis: Application to Clinical Practice*, 8th edn. New York: JB Lippincott.

Carson, V.B. (1989) *Spiritual Dimensions of Nursing Practice*. Philadelphia: WB Saunders.

Cobb, M. (1998) 'Assessing spiritual needs: an examination of practice.' In M. Cobb and V. Robshaw (eds) (1998) *The Spiritual Challenge of Health Care*, 105–118. Edinburgh: Churchill Livingstone.

Cobb, M. (2001) *The Dying Soul: Spiritual Care at the End of Life*. Buckingham: Open University Press.

Cobb, M. and Robshaw, V. (eds) (1998) *The Spiritual Challenge of Health Care*. Edinburgh: Churchill Livingstone.

Colliton, M.A. (1981) 'The spiritual dimension of nursing.' In I.L. Beland and J.Y. Passos (eds) *Clinical Nursing*, 492–501, 4th edn. New York: Macmillan.

Coyle, J. (2002) 'Spirituality and health: towards a framework for exploring the relationship between spirituality and health.' *Journal of Advanced Nursing 37*, 6, 589–597.

Culliford, L. (2002) 'Spiritual care and psychiatric treatment – an introduction.' *Advanced Psychiatric Treatment 8*, 249–260.

Dickinson, C. (1975) 'The search for spiritual meaning.' *American Journal of Nursing 75*, 10, 1789–1793.

Dossey, L. (1993) *Healing Words: The Power of Prayer and the Practice of Medicine*. San Francisco: Harper.

Dunn, P.M. (1993) 'An investigation into the concept of spiritual needs of hospitalised patients, from a nursing perspective.' Unpublished dissertation, Hull: Institute of Nursing Studies, University of Hull.

Ellison, W. (1983) 'Spiritual wellbeing: conceptualisation and measurement.' *Journal of Psychology and Theology 11*, 4, 330–340.

Erikson, H.H. (1963) *Childhood and Society*, 2nd edn. New York: WW Norton.

Farmer, E.S. (ed.) (1996) *Exploring the Spiritual Dimension of Care*. Wiltshire: Quay Books.

Frankl, V.E. (1987) *Man's Search for Meaning: An Introduction to Logotherapy*. London: Hodder and Stoughton.

Harrison, J. (1993) 'Spirituality and nursing practice.' *Journal of Clinical Nursing 2*, 211–217.

Harrison, J. and Burnard, P. (1993) *Spirituality and Nursing Practice*. Aldershot: Avebury.

Henery, N. (2003) 'Constructions of spirituality in contemporary nursing theory.' *Journal of Advanced Nursing 42*, 550–557.

Highfield, M.F. and Cason, C. (1983) 'Spiritual needs of patients: are they recognized?' *Cancer Nursing* (June), 187–192.

Hungelmann, J., Rossi-Kenkel, E., Klassen, L. and Stollenwerk, R.M. (1985) 'Spiritual well being in older adults: harmonious interconnectedness.' *Journal of Religion and Health 24*, 2, 147–153.

Jewell, A. (1998) *Spirituality and Ageing.* London: Jessica Kingsley Publishers.

Jewell, A. (2003) *Ageing, Spirituality and Well-being.* London: Jessica Kingsley Publishers.

Koenig, H.G. (2002) *Spirituality in Patient Care: Why, How, When and What?* Radnor, Pennsylvania: Templeton Foundation Press.

Koenig, H.G., McCullough, M.E. and Larson, D.B. (2001) *Handbook of Religion and Health.* Oxford: Oxford University Press.

Labun, E. (1988) 'Spiritual care: an element in nursing care planning.' *Journal of Advanced Nursing 13*, 314–320.

Leggieri, J. (1986) 'Pastoral care in the hospital: uniqueness and contribution.' *Topics in Clinical Nursing 8*, 2, 47–55.

MacLaren, J. (2004) 'A kaleidoscope of understandings: spiritual nursing in a multi-faith society.' *Journal of Advanced Nursing 45*, 5, 457–462.

MacKinlay, E. (2001) *The Spiritual Dimensions of Ageing.* London: Jessica Kingsley Publishers.

McSherry, W. (1996) 'Raising the spirits.' *Nursing Times 92*, 3, 48–49.

McSherry, W. (2000) *Making Sense of Spirituality in Nursing Practice: An Interactive Approach.* Edinburgh: Churchill Livingstone.

McSherry, W. (2004) 'The meaning of spirituality and spiritual care: an investigation of health care professionals', patients' and public's perceptions.' Unpublished PhD thesis. Leeds: Leeds Metropolitan University.

McSherry, W. and Cash, K. (2004) 'The language of spirituality: an emerging taxonomy.' *International Journal of Nursing Studies 41*, 151–161.

McSherry, W. and Draper, P. (1998) 'The debates emerging from the literature surrounding the concept of spirituality as applied to nursing.' *Journal of Advanced Nursing 27*, 683–691.

Morberg, D.O. (1971) 'Spiritual well-being: background and issues.' White House Conference on Aging, Washington, DC.

Morberg, D.O. (1979) *Spiritual Well-being: Sociological Perspectives.* Washington, DC: University Press of America.

Morrison, R. (1989) 'Spiritual health care and the nurse.' *Nursing Standard 4*, 13/14, 28–29.

Murray, R.B. and Zentner, J.B. (1989) *Nursing Concepts for Health Promotion.* London: Prentice Hall.

Narayanasamy, A. (1991) *Spiritual Care: A Resource Guide.* Lancaster: Quay Books.

Narayanasamy, A. (2001) *Spiritual Care: A Practical Guide for Nurses and Health Care Practitioners*, 2nd edn. Wiltshire: Quay Publishing.

Nash, M. and Stewart, B. (2002) *Spirituality and Social Care Contributing to Personal and Community Well-being.* London: Jessica Kingsley Publishers.

Neuman, B. (1995) *The Neuman Systems Model*, 3rd edn. Norwalk: Appleton and Lange.

Orchard, H. (ed.) (2001) *Spirituality in Health Care Contexts.* London: Jessica Kingsley Publishers.

Pearsall, J. (ed.) (1998) *The New Oxford English Dictionary.* Oxford: Clarendon Press.

Rassool, H.G. (2000) 'The crescent of Islam: healing, nursing and the spiritual dimension: some considerations towards an understanding of the Islamic perspectives on caring.' *Journal of Advanced Nursing 32,* 6, 1476–1484.

Reed, P.G. (1987) 'Spirituality and well-being in terminally-ill hospitalised adults.' *Research in Nursing and Health 10,* 335–344.

Reed, P.G. (1992) 'An emerging paradigm for the investigation of spirituality in nursing.' *Research in Nursing and Health 15,* 349–357.

Robinson, S., Kendrick, K. and Brown, A. (2003) *Spirituality and the Practice of Healthcare.* Houndsmill: Palgrave Macmillan.

Ross, L. (1997) *Nurses' Perceptions of Spiritual Care.* Aldershot: Avebury.

Rumbold, B. (2002) *Spirituality and Palliative Care.* Melbourne, Australia: Oxford University Press.

Shelly, J.A. and Fish, S. (1988) *Spiritual Care: The Nurse's Role,* 3rd edn. Illinois: Inter Varsity Press.

Shirahama, K. and Inoue, E.M. (2001) 'Spirituality in nursing from a Japanese perspective.' *Holistic Nursing Practice 15,* 3, 63–72.

Smith, J. and McSherry, W. (2004) 'Spirituality and child development: a concept analysis.' *Journal of Advanced Nursing 45,* 3, 307–315.

Stallwood, J. and Stoll, R. (1975) 'Spiritual dimensions of nursing practice.' In I.L. Beland and J.Y. Passos (eds) *Clinical Nursing,* 3rd edn. New York: Macmillan.

Stanworth, R. (2004) *Recognizing Spiritual Needs in People who are Dying.* Oxford: Oxford University Press.

Stoll, R.I. (1989) 'The essence of spirituality.' In V.B. Carson (ed.) *Spiritual Dimensions of Nursing Practice.* Philadelphia: WB Saunders.

Stoter, D.J. (1995) *Spiritual Aspects of Health Care.* London: Mosby.

Sulmasy, D.P. (1997) *The Healer's Calling: A Spirituality for Physicians and Other Health Care Professionals.* New York: Paulist Press.

Swinton, J. (2001) *Spirituality and Mental Health Care: Rediscovering a 'Forgotten' Dimension.* London: Jessica Kingsley Publishers.

Tanyi, R.A. (2002) 'Towards clarification of the meaning of spirituality.' *Journal of Advanced Nursing 39,* 5, 500–509.

Taylor, E.J. (2002) *Spiritual Care, Nursing Theory, Research and Practice.* New Jersey: Prentice Hall.

Travelbee, J. (1966) *Interpersonal Aspects of Nursing.* Philadelphia, PA: Davis.

Turner, P. (1996) 'Caring more, doing less.' *Nursing Times 92,* 34, 59–60.

Walsh, M. and Ford, P. (1989) *Nursing Rituals: Research and Rational Actions.* Oxford: Heinemann Nursing.

Willows, D. and Swinton, J. (2000) *Spiritual Dimensions of Pastoral Care: Practical Theology in a Multidisciplinary Context.* London: Jessica Kingsley Publishers.

Wright, M.C. (2001) 'Chaplaincy in hospice and hospital: findings from a survey in England and Wales.' *Palliative Medicine 15*, 229–242.

Wright, M.C. (2002) 'The Essence of spiritual care: a phenomenological enquiry.' *Palliative Medicine 16*, 125–132.

Wright, S. (1997) 'Free the spirit.' *Nursing Times 93*, 17, 28–29.

Further reading

Exploring the meaning of the word spirituality

These articles look specifically at the meaning of the word 'spirituality' and will help develop your knowledge and understanding of the concept.

Bash, A. (2004) 'Spirituality: the emperor's new clothes.' *Journal of Clinical Nursing 13*, 1, 11–16.

Cawley, N. (1997) 'An exploration of the concept of spirituality.' *International Journal of Palliative Care 3*, 1, 31–36.

Henery, N. (2003) 'The reality of visions: contemporary theories of spirituality in social work.' *British Journal of Social Work 33*, 1105–1113.

MacLaren, J. (2004) 'A kaleidoscope of understandings: spiritual nursing in a multi-faith society.' *Journal of Advanced Nursing 45*, 5, 457–462.

McSherry, W. and Cash, K. (2004) 'The language of spirituality: an emerging taxonomy.' *International Journal of Nursing Studies 41*, 151–161.

Narayanasamy, A. (2004) 'Commentary on MacLaren, J. (2004) A kaleidoscope of understandings: spiritual nursing in a multi-faith society.' *Journal of Advanced Nursing 45*, 5, 457–464.

Explaining the relationship between different religions and spirituality

These authors discuss in some detail the influences that different religions have had on society and implications for health care.

Henley, A. and Schott, J. (1999) *Culture, Religion and Patient Care in a Multi-Ethnic Society.* London: Age Concern.

Markham, I. (1998) 'Spirituality and the world faiths.' In M. Cobb and V. Robshaw (1998) *The Spiritual Challenge of Health Care*, 73–87. Edinburgh: Churchill Livingstone.

Narayanasamy, A. (2001) *Spiritual Care: A Practical Guide for Nurses and Health Care Practitioners*, 2nd edn, 37–72. Wiltshire: Quay Publishing.

Rassool, H.G. (2000) 'The crescent of Islam: healing, nursing and the spiritual dimension: some considerations towards an understanding of the Islamic perspectives on caring.' *Journal of Advanced Nursing 32*, 6, 1476–1484.

Sheikh, A. and Gatrad, A.R. (2000) *Caring for Muslim Patients.* Oxon: Radcliffe Medical Press.

Taylor, E.J. (2002) *Spiritual Care, Nursing Theory, Research and Practice,* 103–136, 228–261. New Jersey: Prentice Hall.

General reading

Any of the books identified in Box 2.1 and listed in the references will provide you with an insight into the concept of spirituality and health care. You may want to select one from your own profession to browse.

3

Spirituality Within the Context of Holism

Introduction

This chapter explores the place that spirituality has within the context of holism. The adjective holistic is used frequently within the caring professions without taking into account its implications. However, consideration needs to be given to what we mean by holism and how the concept may need to be revised to accommodate changing theory and practice. These debates are presented and examined against the emerging literature surrounding spirituality and the provision of spiritual care. The place that spirituality has within the context of theories and models is briefly discussed.

Activity 3.1

Spend several minutes reflecting upon the terms holism and holistic. Write down any thoughts or ideas that come to mind. Think about how you were introduced to these terms and how frequently you hear these words being used in your practice area.

The terms holism and holistic care are used frequently by health care professionals. Your reflections may have revealed that these terms are associated with treating the 'whole' person, or providing care that seeks to address all the dimensions of an individual's life – for example, the physical, social, psychological and spiritual (Box 3.1).

Box 3.1 The four aspects of holism

Biological

This refers to the physical and biological process or function of an individual essential to maintain life.

Psychological

Usually implies the cognitive, intellectual, emotional aspects of the individual that may shape personality and mental functioning.

Social

The cultural norms, values and beliefs that influence and classify individuals into different groups or communities.

Spiritual

A vague term used normally to indicate an individual's inner beliefs commonly related to religious affiliation or belief in the existence of a God or supreme power.

You were probably introduced to these terms during your health care training or education. Alternatively, you may have heard the words being used in practice or read them incorporated within a philosophy of care or academic textbook.

If you had been asked to draw a diagram that represents holism, then you may well have drawn one similar to Figure 3.1.

The circle in Figure 3.1 represents the 'whole' person while the four different quarters, described in Box 3.1, represent fundamental dimensions. However, this could be classified as a reductionist approach because there is no indication that all four quarters or dimensions are interrelated or dependent upon each other. The diagram reduces the whole into manageable mechanistic units. The diagrammatic representation is void of any interaction or interconnection between the individual, his or her environment or other

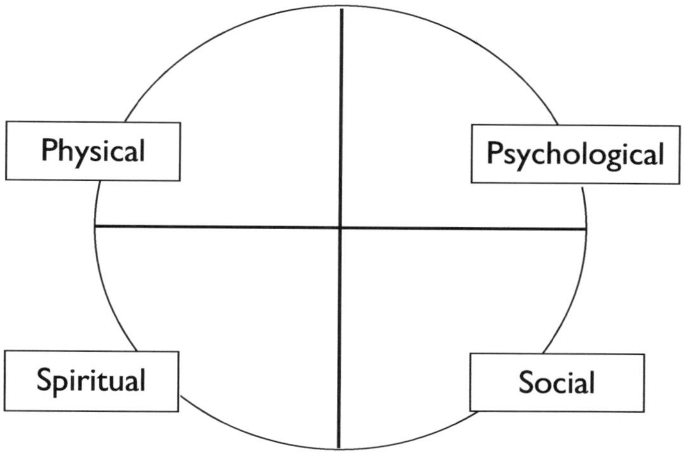

Figure 3.1: A common representation of holism

people – indeed the whole of creation. It assumes that individuals function in isolation. Each aspect of our being is placed in a functional box not overlapping the next (as shown by the black solid lines). Holism is represented in a very narrow insular way. This raises two important questions:

- What is holism?
- How has the concept been defined within health care?

Holism

The word 'holism' originates from the Greek word 'holos', meaning whole (Griffin 1993; Ham-Ying 1993). The term holism implies that all dimensions of our lives are equally important to our functioning and well-being: 'The whole is greater than the sum of its parts' (Patterson 1998). Yet your reflection reveals that the biological and medical models of care contradict the term since they separate individuals into functional mechanistic units or biological systems (discussed in Chapter 1), often at the expense of seeing the whole person and his or her situation (see Box 3.2).

Several authors (Buckle 1993; Griffin 1993; Kolcaba 1997; Paley 2002; Patterson 1998; Thorne 2001) have explored and discussed the term holism, and their conclusions indicate there may be no single definition because the term is vague and difficult to pin down.

Ham-Ying (1993) implies that nurses do not have an adequate understanding of the concept of holism, nor a sufficient educational preparation, and the result may be that holistic care will not be fully operational within the context of nursing practice. With this point in mind, it might be useful to discuss how the term is defined within nursing.

The Churchill Livingstone (1996, p.176) *Dictionary of Nursing* does not offer a definition of holism but defines holistic as: 'In a nursing context, caring for the whole patient – total patient care.'

Box 3.2 Definitions of holism, holistic and reductionism

Holism

The individual is perceived as a 'whole'. There is acknowledgement that no systems – biological, psychosocial, spiritual or environmental – can be viewed in isolation because they all 'make up the whole person'.

Holistic

Attending to all dimensions of an individual with equal importance.

Reductionism

The tendency to reduce or divide individuals into functional mechanist units. This is the opposite of holism.

This definition reinforces the notion that holistic care concerns the entire person. A possible reason why these terms are open to misinterpretation is because, like spirituality, a great deal of uncertainty still surrounds them. Buckle (1993) argues that the term holism is used inaccurately because it is used interchangeably with the word complementary, thus underlining the confusion and misconceptions surrounding the use of the term. From this brief analysis of the term holism, it would appear that there is some degree of ambiguity about the precise meaning of the word. Despite these uncertainties, the relevance and benefits of using these terms in the provision of health and nursing care cannot be dismissed. Holism is a common feature in many nursing models (Pearson, Vaughan and Fitzgerald 2005), and has guided and shaped the direction of nursing care throughout its inception and evolution.

In summary, the word holism is used to describe the 'whole' and the adjective holistic is used to describe the application of the term to practice –

for example, the provision of holistic care. There is recognition that all parts of an individual share equal importance in a balanced manner. If we are providing holistic care, then we attend to all dimensions of an individual, giving each the same amount of importance.

Reductionism

A reductionist approach would be to reduce the individual into manageable units. From within my own professional discipline, the Roper, Logan and Tierney (1980) nursing model could be classified as a reductionist model because it divides the individual into a set of systems or activities that are required for daily living, such as breathing, elimination, eating and drinking, and sexuality. These types of approach to case management have been adopted within other professional groups to aid assessment and diagnosis. Yet the reality in the systems highlighted is that all these systems are related to and dependent upon each other. A purely reductionist approach focuses upon specific aspects of the person without giving due consideration to the other dimensions and their relationships with each other. However, clinical experience shows that there may be some benefits from implementing a reductionist approach. Different aspects of care can be delegated and managed by the appropriate professionals. It would appear that this approach to patient management is used in many health care settings. This is illustrated by the following Case study 3.1.

Case study 3.1 A case for reductionism

A middle-aged man with Type I diabetes mellitus is admitted with a 'diabetic foot'. He has a large ulcer affecting his right big toe and is unable to cope at home with his illness. The man complains that his life has been altered dramatically by the condition.

Activity 3.2

Spend several minutes reflecting upon this man's situation and write down how a reductionist approach might address the problems of the diabetic foot and other issues the man is experiencing.

The chances are that you identified a number of professionals who may be asked to contribute to this man's care needs (Box 3.3).

Box 3.3 How reductionism addresses the 'whole' – achieving total patient care

Doctors	Overall management of medical care
Nurses	Overall responsibility for nursing care interventions
Dietician	Nutritional support
Podiatrist	Management of diabetic foot
Occupational therapist	Adaptation and adjustment in activities of living
Religious/spiritual leader	Religious and spiritual needs
Social worker	Advice on support services available
Physiotherapist	Mobility
Diabetes specialist nurse	Advice concerning management of diabetes

Closer inspection of the list reveals how reductionism delegates areas of responsibility to other professionals. It could still be said that the man is receiving 'holistic care' or total patient care, because the key aspects are being addressed. Problems with this approach are that a breakdown in communication can mean that important information is not communicated. Likewise, professionals may only focus upon their own specific areas of responsibility, which can sometimes mean that problems the patient may have remain undetected. The greatest danger is that care can appear fragmented and an holistic perspective of how the different dimensions affect and are affected by each other is lost. Some practice areas remove this risk by holding multidisciplinary or case conferences where information is exchanged, progress discussed and further interventions decided.

Models of health care: A brief overview

It is not the intention of this chapter to provide a detailed analysis of all the health care or indeed the nursing models that have been developed; that is beyond the scope of this book. This section will look at the place that spirituality has within some of these models, demonstrating how the growing awareness of the importance of spirituality to an individual's sense of well-being has led some theorists to revisit and revise their theories to incorporate the spiritual dimension. An example of this in nursing would be Neuman (1995).

Activity 3.3

Spend some time reflecting upon any health care model that you have heard about or that you use or have used in your practice. Write down your understanding of the model, paying particular attention to any aspect of spirituality that it might address.

Undertaking Activity 3.3 may have proved difficult for two main reasons. First, our knowledge of health care is dependent upon two fundamental factors:

1. The models we have been introduced to during our training or programme of education. Related to this is the manner in which they were taught and applied to practice. Often if they are taught very theoretically and not applied you can be left more confused, finding it difficult to see the relevance of such material.
2. The regularity with which we use or encounter such models within practice.

Second, within nursing in the UK and perhaps this may apply to other professional groups, we are normally introduced to a small range of theories and models. It could be argued that the teaching of health care theories and models is purely an academic exercise. The relevance of such knowledge received may not be directly relevant to one's area of practice (unless the area in which we work uses the particular model[s] being presented as a framework for care delivery). Therefore, within the UK, you may only have educational and practical experience in the use of the 'model of daily living' because this has been developed by British nurse theorists and is widely acknowledged and used in clinical practice.

What is a model?

A model represents a personal view of how individuals are made, function and interact with the world. Walsh (1991, p.8), discussing nursing models, summarizes these as:

> Nursing models, therefore, are not watertight theories, but rather sets of ideas about the way patients and nurses interact. The dangers of reductionism and losing touch with reality are such that model development must take place with at least one foot in the real world of practical nursing care.

Therefore, models represent the world of nursing or health care from different perspectives, offering a set of ideas or a framework for the delivery of care. Conceptual models of nursing and health care present a set of ideas concerning the way that individuals may live, react to illness or interact with their world. It must be stressed that they represent only one world view. For example, Orem's (1985) theories concerning self-care or Neuman's (1995) systems model address the different systems involved in people's reaction to health and illness. It could even be argued that there are as many nursing and health care models as there are thinking professionals, since we all have our own individual and personal philosophies concerning what makes us think, feel and react differently to stressful situations.

These points bring into question the direct relevance and purpose of nursing models in the delivery of nursing. Walsh (1991) believes nursing models are useful because they provide structure and direction in the provision of care, while other authors are very sceptical and critical of their relevance to nursing (Cash 1990; Draper 1990; Kenny 1993; Luker 1988). Despite recent criticism of nursing models (Tierney 1998), it would appear that they are here to stay.

Spirituality and health care models

It was stated earlier that the majority of health care and in particular nursing models embrace a holistic approach. If this statement were accurate, then such models by their very nature should address the concept of spirituality explicitly within their theories and frameworks. Recent debates indicate that this is not the case and only a minority of health care, and from within my own profession, nursing models incorporate or address the spiritual nature of individuals. Oldnall (1995, p.418) provides some reasons why the spiritual dimension is not adequately addressed within nursing and these arguments could be extended to include all health care theories:

> Perhaps one reason why many conceptual and theoretical models and theories do not appear to work in clinical practice is because they have evolved in the echelons of academia and have been devolved down to the practitioners to operationalize at a clinical level. This may explain, to some degree, why the concept of spirituality has been omitted totally, or at least not developed sufficiently, in existing theories and models.

Oldnall implies that the assumption that most nursing models have an holistic approach to care is inaccurate and misguided. If nursing models and theories embraced holism, then they would address the spiritual dimension. Oldnall (1995, 1996) implies that there needs to be a cultural shift – a change in emphasis. Models should not be solely developed in the 'ivory towers of academia' and then expected to work in practice. This top-down approach to theory development may overlook and fail to incorporate many issues that are being faced by health care professionals working on the front line. This approach may have prevented the spiritual dimension from being incorporated within contemporary health care theories and models.

It appears that the academic era of health care is being challenged within the UK, and that the change in emphasis that has been sought by chief nurses and those in practice has arrived. In the mid-1980s, there was a move to improve the educational and professional credibility of nursing and, through a recent quality initiative, the education and preparation of all health care professions by integrating their education within universities. This initiative took place before other health professions were already located within higher education. However, recent discontent and levels of dissatisfaction among managers in health and social services have resulted in a change of opinion.

For example, in the government's document *Making a Difference: Strengthening the Nursing, Midwifery and Health Visiting Contribution to Health and Health Care* (Department of Health 1999), the need for education and practice to work more closely in the education and training of student nurses was emphasized. The pendulum has swung (at the right too much emphasis on academia, and at the left signalling an all apprentice style of learning with no academic recognition) too far to the right, and it would seem that NHS Trusts and the voice and concerns of the consumer now have a greater say in the education of all health care professionals. This approach is of particular importance to matters concerning spirituality and the provision of spiritual care.

Importantly, this shift in emphasis must be reflected in subsequent theory development. There is a need to have a 'bottom-up' approach whereby practice is put into theory, or theories and models will remain detached from practice and in the realm of academics or theorists.

CAUTION

If the concerns of those in practice relating to this dimension of care are not listened to, then any attempt to develop this aspect of care will remain an academic exercise unrelated to and divorced from the reality of practice.

What do the theorists have to say? In addition, what can we learn from them?

I have deliberately not revised this section, and left the focus upon nursing theorists; the rationale for this is that, first, many of the points raised in this section have implications for the whole of health care. Second, a review of the health care literature concerning spirituality demonstrates that all health care professions are learning from the debate and knowledge developed within each other's disciplines, transferring and adapting such knowledge to meet their own specific practices.

Martsolf and Mickley (1998) present a review of modern nurse theorists' ideas concerning spirituality. After reviewing the contribution to nursing knowledge made by some of the contemporary nurse theorists, Martsolf and Mickley indicate the position that spirituality has within those ideas. This section offers a summary of the information provided in Martsolf and Mickley (1998). It is beyond the scope of this book to provide a full critique of the place spirituality holds within each model. Therefore, this section will only indicate whether the model addresses the spiritual dimension explicitly or implicitly (as defined in Box 3.4) and provide a very brief outline of how spirituality is addressed by a particular theorist (Boxes 3.5 and 3.6).

Box 3.4 The terms defined

Explicitly

There is clear mention or reference to the importance of the concept. Removal of the spiritual element would have an impact upon the theory.

Implicitly

Reference to the spiritual dimension is inferred in the theories and concepts of the model or addressed as a subcomponent. However, removal of the spiritual element would have no influence on the theory.

Box 3.5 Spirituality implicit within the theory or model

Johnson (1980)
The 'behavioural systems' model indicates that we have a specific set of response patterns that act together to form an integrated whole. The behavioural system comprises several subsystems. It is within these subsystems that spirituality may feature. One subsystem is affiliation – the need to relate to one's own beliefs such as the belief in a God.

Leininger (1991, 2001)
The concepts of 'cultural care theory' are central to Leininger's work. It could be argued that spirituality is loosely addressed in connection with the religious influences upon which different cultures are formed.

Levine (1967)
This model has 'four conservation principles' and considers that we are adaptive beings in a state of interaction with our environment, both inner and external. The external environment consists of three key components: perceptual, operational and conceptual. It is within the conceptual that reference is made to spirituality.

Rogers (1980)
This model considers 'unitary human beings'. The word spirituality was not used directly in the work addressing the science of unitary human beings, but has been attached to aspects of the theory by other authors (Smith 1994).

Roper et al. (1990)
Early editions of *The Elements of Nursing* did not give recognition to the spiritual dimension. However, by the third edition, there is realization of the place that spirituality may have with regard to the well-being of individuals. Spirituality is not addressed explicitly but rather within the context of religion and culture (Bradshaw 1994).

Roy (1980)
Called the 'adaptation model', this model considers the moral, ethical and spiritual self. This aspect of Roy's model helps the individual to answer questions in relation to belief and existence.

Many nurse theorists acknowledge the place that spirituality has within the context of holism. Whether the spiritual dimension is explicit or implicit within the theory, this indicates a growing realization of the importance of the dimension to a sense of well-being and completeness. The models reinforce the need for the spiritual dimension to be considered in both an individual and a global sense.

The spirituality of an individual is influenced and shaped by many factors: environmental, internal, political and social. To view spirituality purely as a theory in its own right would be divisive and reductionist. There is a need to be aware of the many systems and forces, both positive and negative, that can shape an individual's sense of health and total well-being. The theories and models indicate that individuals are made up of many systems interacting with each other. These systems work in harmony to maintain equilibrium. Many forces or stressors can affect the individual's state. These forces can be internal or external. It is the individual's ability to adapt or restore balance when affected by such forces that results in illness or restoration to wholeness. The health care professional's role is to assist in this process of restoration. If restoration cannot be achieved, then their role may be to prepare the individual for a dignified death.

Box 3.6 Spirituality explicit within the theory/model

Neuman (1995)
The 'Neuman's systems model' includes the spiritual variable. Neuman indicates that the patient may not have a conscious awareness of this component but it is present in all individuals. The spiritual variable has the potential to influence individuals' systems positively. Spiritual awareness may be developed at any time during the lifespan.

Newman (1986)
Newman's 'model of health' assumes that health is associated with the expansion of an individual's consciousness. Spirituality is used broadly in connection with human interactions.

Parse (1981)
In the Man-living-health theory, the term spirituality is not used. However, one of the theoretical principles of this theory is that individuals can choose personal meaning. Therefore, if the concept were removed from Parse's theory, the work would be adversely affected.

Watson (1985)
This philosophy and science of human caring operates around nurse and patient interactions. The spiritual dimension of the individual is acknowledged. The goal of nursing is to enable individuals to achieve a balance between mind, body and spirit, finding meaning in their existence.

The theorists' work highlights the complex nature of human organisms and how we are interdependent and interconnected with others, the wider community and ourselves. Nursing theories and health care models alert us to the fact that spirituality is an integral aspect of the individual's lived, total experience. It operates and pervades all levels of an individual's existence from the cradle to the grave. The theories reveal that the spiritual dimension is important at behavioural levels – our interactions with the environment and others. It is concerned with each person's ability to find meaning and purpose in situations and events. It enables us to achieve or reach our optimum potential.

Those nursing and health care theories and models that omit the spiritual dimension are failing to address a fundamental concept. The omission fails to recognize the impact that a loss of spiritual well-being might have on the overall quality of life and sense of well-being experienced by an individual. The absence of the spiritual dimension may not be a conscious omission but rather a preoccupation with the political, economic, educational and social influences that prevailed at the time of construction. The absence of spirituality within some models may reflect the theorists' inability to appreciate or critically appraise material used in their theory development. Bradshaw (1994, p.188) shares this view:

> But this analysis has also highlighted a further problem in nursing theory. That is, not only do nursing theories uncritically incorporate concepts from other academic disciplines without reference to their philosophical background, context, and coherence, but they also employ insights and arguments from fellow nurses without critically examining or even addressing the source of their positions.

Interestingly, this argument is directed towards an attempt by Roper *et al.* (1990) to address the concept of spirituality within their model of nursing. The point reinforces the need for theorists to appraise critically existing knowledge before incorporating it within subsequent revision.

This brief review of theories and models indicates that the spiritual dimension has an important place within the context of holism. The spiritual dimension, as represented in several of the nursing theories, seems to be a force that brings unity and harmony to the human state.

Box 3.7 Food for thought

Before academics, and indeed practitioners, accuse theorists who fail to acknowledge the spiritual dimension of being misguided and lacking spiritual awareness, we must consider the full picture. It may be the era and social context in which theories are constructed and tested that determines individuals' thinking and assumptions. It will be interesting to review health care theories that are currently being constructed in a time of spiritual reawakening.

Spirituality as a unifying force

In Chapter 2, the analogy of spirituality as a football was made, stressing that it is a force that pervades, integrates and interconnects all aspects of our existence and being. It has been suggested in the previous section that spirituality is a force that brings unity and stability to our being. Surveying nurse perceptions of spirituality, McSherry (1997, p.120) writes:

> Of the nurses surveyed (276) 50.3 per cent felt that spirituality was a unifying force which enabled individuals to be at peace with oneself and the world. This finding was reinforced when McSherry (2004) interviewed a range of health care professionals, again many of the nurses described spirituality as originating from within themselves (something innate) a force which brings unity and harmony. These findings imply that nurses in particular were aware that spirituality is multi-dimensional which is related to the natural and supernatural dimensions of existence. These would be the Vertical and Horizontal dimensions as defined by Stoll (1989).

McSherry's (2004) research findings suggest that health care professionals and some patients perceive spirituality as something that influences the physical, psychological and social aspects of our being in an integrated manner. Spirituality is an invisible force that brings unity and harmony to self, others and the larger universe. The spiritual dimension is a mysterious and transcendent force that assists the individual in finding meaning, purpose and fulfilment. It is a force that transcends the rational and intellectual capabilities of our human state, uniting us with the whole of creation both at a material and supernatural level.

Models representing the spiritual dimension

Stoll (1989) uses a two-dimensional approach to show the relationship between the spiritual dimension and other aspects of our lives (Figure 3.2). She uses a vertical line to show the individual's connection with the mystical-transcendental domain. This relationship may consist of a belief in a supreme being or God. The supreme being may be values or principles that guide the person's life. A horizontal line is used to describe the relationship that exists between self and others. An inner circle is used to depict the person and his or her relationship with both vertical and horizontal dimensions. Stoll stresses the interrelatedness and interconnectedness of all the dimensions by the use of dashed lines. Three spiritual needs operating within the model are the needs for love, forgiveness and trust. For Stoll, spirituality is developed throughout life and the dimension may come into focus during times of health and illness.

One major limitation of this approach is that it separates the different dimensions. For example, the vertical line representing the mystical is not

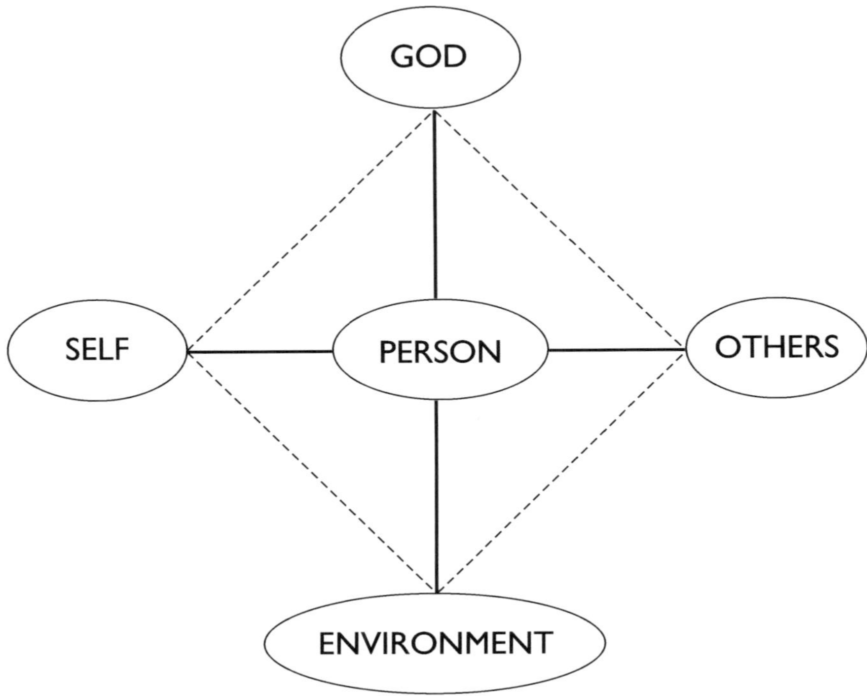

Figure 3.2: Stoll's two-dimensional model (adapted from Stoll 1989, p.8)

integrated with the psychosocial or environmental. The model does not seem to stress the unifying nature and intimacy that spirituality has with all the different aspects of a person's life. The model could be described as dualistic and functionalist because it implies that spirituality serves a specific need – for example, the need for love, trust and forgiveness (McSherry and Draper 1998; Shelly and Fish 1988). If these needs are met, then the person will have meaning, purpose and fulfilment in life.

In Chapter 2, the 'conceptual model of the nature of man' described by Stallwood and Stoll (1975) was mentioned. This model, illustrated in Figure 3.3, emphasizes the integrated nature of individuals and illustrates clearly the place that spirituality has within the context of holism. Unlike Stoll's two-dimensional approach, this model represents simply the relationship between the physical, psychosocial and spiritual, indicating that spirituality expresses itself via the total being.

In this model, the outermost circle represents the physical body – the biological world. This is the body as seen by others and self. The physical body enables individuals to relate to the world via the five main senses of touch, taste, hearing, sight and smell. The second circle depicts the psychosocial dimension. This is the part of the person associated with self-consciousness, personality, intellect, moral senses and will. It could be argued that the

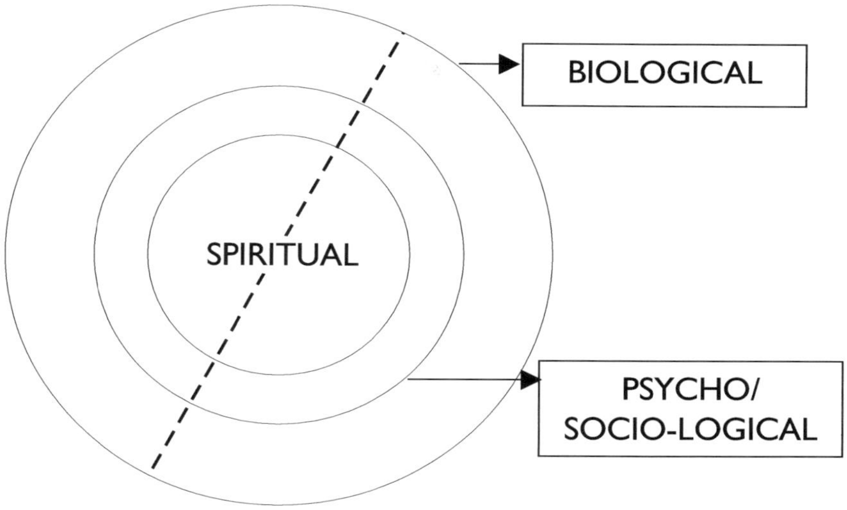

Figure 3.3: Stallwood and Stoll's (1975) conceptual model of the nature of humans (Beland and Passos 1975, p.1087)

psychological aspects are influenced and shaped by the social context and environmental and cultural influences. The innermost circle is described as spiritual. It is hard to define and comprehend and is therefore mysterious. The spirit pervades all other dimensions of the individual. Within the spiritual realm is the potential for awareness of God – however that is defined by the individual. The inner circle represents the vertical line in Stoll's two-dimensional model. The broken lines in the diagram indicate that individuals function as a 'whole'.

The physical body (outer circle) influences the psychosocial and spiritual dimensions. The psychosocial (second circle) expresses itself through the physical, while the spiritual pervades every aspect of an individual's total being. In essence the human spirit unifies the whole person.

The way in which all these dimensions are interconnected and interdependent are illustrated by Case study 3.2. The case study illustrates how the different circles are all interrelated and interconnected. James had begun to experience physical symptoms as a result of the unrest and loss of stability in the spiritual and psychosocial domains. The sense of guilt he experienced was disrupting the flow of energy and stability in all aspects of his life. The cumulative effect of his addiction was the manifestation of depression accompanied by nausea and vomiting. James' entire being had been affected by the spiritual, psychosocial stressors. This case study illustrates simply Stallwood and Stoll's (1975) conceptual model of the nature of humans.

Case study 3.2 A sense of guilt

James is 47 years of age. He was admitted onto an acute psychiatric admissions unit for depression resulting in weight loss for which no pathology had been diagnosed. On admission he looked very anxious and withdrawn. He communicated with staff as a matter of courtesy but did not really identify or relate to any other patients on the unit. The admitting nurse found it difficult to assess James' mental status. He used one-word answers and did not really disclose much about himself or the recent problems that he had been experiencing. His entire body language used closed postures – indicating further his reluctance for anyone to come close. James has been married for 20 years and his wife cannot comprehend the change in personality that he is displaying. Several months earlier they had a loving and open relationship. Several days passed and James appeared more relaxed and less threatened by his admission into the unit. He started to communicate more easily with all staff and other patients on the unit.

In the course of a conversation with one of the nurses, James disclosed the source of his anxiety. He recalled that several years earlier a friend had introduced him to the gambling circuit. In recent months, the friend had been threatening to reveal James' hidden secret to his wife. Since this revelation, James had been unable to sleep. He had become preoccupied with the repercussions of this upon his marriage and family. Now he felt very guilty and anxious about the entire situation, becoming increasingly depressed. As the months passed and the blackmail intensified, he felt more trapped and isolated. Eventually he met the ransom by paying the friend several thousand pounds – severing his ties with gambling and the friend in an attempt to preserve his relationships.

A limitation of the Stallwood and Stoll model is the over-preoccupation with the intellectual and moral cognitive functioning of the individual. The model implies that a functioning intellect is a necessity to the development of spirituality. This issue is explored further in the next section.

Biological basis?

Narayanasamy (1999) reviewed the work of Hardy (1979) and others – for example, Hay (1994) – revisiting the notion that there is growing evidence to support the biological basis or origin for spirituality. This biological basis is based on the evolutionary principle of 'biological survival value'. This work has now been extended by the emergence of neurological work (Newberg *et al.* 2002) and neuro-theology, a science concerned with the identification and labeling of specific areas within the brain that are associated with the manifestation of a sense of transcendence.

Activity 3.4

Spend several minutes reflecting upon the two different models presented in this section. Write down any thoughts, ideas or concerns that you might have about spirituality and holism.

Psychological and spiritual

When I am presenting workshops or lectures concerning spirituality, one question that is continually asked is: How do you distinguish the spiritual from the psychological?

My immediate response is to sigh and take a deep breath before attempting to offer an explanation or an illustration. However, this question is extremely important and worthy of further explanation. It is true that many of the things associated with spirituality, such as our need to find meaning, purpose and fulfilment, are directly related to our psychological well-being. The danger is to reduce and separate our spiritual needs and psychological needs into different domains or categories. Spirituality is not a separate entity that can be turned on or off at the touch of a switch because it is continually present, whether we are conscious of this or not. This point is highlighted in Case study 3.3.

Case study 3.3 Psychological and spiritual

Martha is 56 years old. At the age of 50, she was diagnosed with pre-senile dementia. The signs and symptoms had been associated with stress. However, a CT scan confirmed organic changes and the diagnosis. Prior to her diagnosis, she had been a highly successful businesswoman. Her final position was director of a large international company. Despite being successful, Martha had a strong belief and faith in a God but did not attend any formal religious organization.

In her spare time, Martha had enjoyed a range of activities such as travel, painting and regular cross-country runs. She liked to spend time on her own reflecting and keeping in touch with the creative aspects of her personality. The slow progression of the disease meant that Martha was very much aware of the deteriorative nature of the illness and the result that this might have upon her life. As the disease progressed, she was unable to maintain her interests and activities. She became withdrawn and isolated within her own inner world. Familiar faces and locations lost their meaning. Martha's modesty and privacy were lost as she began to become incontinent. Her entire personality changed, resulting in aggressive outbursts, and on several occasions household objects were thrown around the room. Martha had become the complete opposite to everything in which she believed.

Having read this case study, you are probably wondering what this has to do with the psychological and spiritual debate. One important question that needs to be asked to help us make sense of this situation is: has Martha's spirituality changed as a result of the progressive disease?

Martha is still the same person with all her personal beliefs and values. What has changed is her psychological functioning and processes. Fundamentally, Martha is still the same individual, but her cognitive processes and physiological functions have been disrupted by this degenerative disorder. It is not the intention of this chapter to enter into deep philosophical debate. However, I would argue that Martha still has the same spirituality and that, even among the inner turmoil, she is a spiritual being who possesses spiritual needs that require spiritual care.

This case study highlights the fact that spirituality pervades all dimensions of one's existence in a meaningful and intricate manner, whether there is a conscious awareness of this or not. Spirituality and the spiritual dimension still exist in the absence of a functioning intellect or other psychological processes (McSherry 2001). This point contradicts Stallwood and Stoll (1975, p.1088), who write: 'An individual may choose which components will be master (god, controlling force) of his person – the body, the intellect, the emotion, the will, the moral sense, or the spirit.'

The same principles implicit in Martha's situation can be applied to individuals with severe learning disabilities or any other condition that affects psychological function or reasoning. Tournier (1954) indicates that the spirit expresses itself through the physical and psychological aspects of our lives but it is neither physical nor psychological. Therefore, we can conclude by saying that spirituality is of another dimension that transcends nature. It is something very mysterious but real. However, caution is required because there is a danger that spirituality is viewed purely in terms of transcendence as Piles (1990, p.38) writes:

> It is necessary that the spiritual dimension be recognized as that part of the human being that seeks to worship someone or something (such as God) outside one's own powers that controls and/or sustains the person especially in a time of crisis.

Therefore, I feel that the spiritual and psychosocial dimensions debate will continue to rumble on. On a final note, does it matter how an individual's needs are classified spiritual or psychosocial so long as such needs are met, as in the case of Martha?

What is the relevance to health care practice?

This chapter has been very abstract in that it has addressed the concepts of holism and spirituality in theoretical and academic terms. The material has probably left you asking yourself a fundamental question: What are the implications of all this for health care practice?

The material presented in this chapter reveals that the concepts of holism and spirituality are very complex and subjective. It would appear that there is no single authoritative definition for either word. The brief exploration of spirituality within the context of health care, theories and models suggests that spirituality is a fundamental part of what makes individuals experience health and an overall sense of well-being. Yet some of the points raised in this chapter warrant further clarification because they have important implications for practice. These points are presented in Box 3.8.

The chapter has demonstrated that there still exists some ambiguity and misconception surrounding the words holism and holistic. When using the term holism, all aspects of an individual must be considered, both micro (concerning the individual) and macro (concerning the wider context such as political, economic and environmental factors). When applying the terms to practice, consideration must be given to more than just the physical, psychological, social and spiritual. A narrow definition does not recognize the interconnectedness or interdependence of the different domains.

Models of nursing and health care demonstrate the uniqueness and complex nature of individuals. However, such theories must incorporate the

Box 3.8 Implications for practice

Ambiguity in definition of holism and spirituality – implications for practice.

Models of health care and the absence of spirituality within them.

Application of theory into practice and vice versa – practice into theory.

A need to generate theory that addresses the spiritual dimension in that it reflects the concerns of practitioners and the public whom we serve.

concerns of those who have to use these models in practice – namely, the practitioner. Theory development must also arise from within practice – instead of being devised and articulated in the realms of academia and thrust upon the practitioner. Practitioners who are directly involved in care delivery are indicating a deficit in some of the models because they do not address the spiritual dimension. Subsequent theory development or revision needs to incorporate these concerns and address the omission. The political drives that have been initiated signal support for the inclusion of the spiritual dimension. There now appears to be a realization that there needs to be a bottom-up and a top-down approach to theory development like the formation of stalactites and stalagmites in a dark cave. The process of integrating theory and practice will only be complete when both can work together, just like the stalactite and stalagmite fusing together. However, the process of fusion in the dark cave will take many decades. The luxury of time is not available to the health care profession because the situation will arise where theory does not reflect practice and vice versa. It is evident that practitioners are aware of the need to attend to individual spiritual needs. This should now be reflected in the content of all health care curricula.

Conclusion

This chapter has demonstrated the place that spirituality has within the context of holism. A brief overview of the place that spirituality has within some health care and nursing models has been provided. However, this analysis is very simplistic and not comprehensive. Yet the information indicates that there is an urgent need for theory and practice to unite. Some of these issues concerning the place of spirituality with the context of holism will rumble on for many more years. It is apparent that spirituality does have an important and central place within human existence. The challenge to the health care professions is to reach a consensus and common vocabulary when addressing the two important issues of holism and spirituality. Perhaps it is even time to draw a line under the 'what constitutes spirituality?' debate and for all health care professionals to engage with the implications and pragmatics of providing spiritual care. Until these debates are settled, the spiritual dimension will remain an elusive, mysterious aspect of human existence.

Box 3.9 Final thought

Do you think a consensus will be reached by theorists and practitioners about the exact role that spirituality plays within people's lives?

References

Bradshaw, A. (1994) *Lighting the Lamp: The Spiritual Dimension of Nursing Care.* London: Scutari Press.

Buckle, J. (1993) 'When is holism not complementary?' *British Journal of Nursing 2,* 15, 744–745.

Cash, K. (1990) 'Nursing models and the idea of nursing.' *International Journal of Nursing Studies 27,* 3, 249–256.

Churchill Livingstone (1996) *Churchill Livingstone's Dictionary of Nursing,* 17th edn. Edinburgh: Churchill Livingstone.

Department of Health (1999) *Making a Difference: Strengthening the Nursing, Midwifery and Health Visiting Contribution to Health and Health Care.* London: Department of Health.

Draper, P. (1990) 'The development of theory in British nursing: current position and future prospects.' *Journal of Advanced Nursing 15,* 12–15.

Griffin, A. (1993) 'Holism in nursing: its meaning and value.' *British Journal of Nursing 2,* 6, 310–312.

Ham-Ying, S. (1993) 'Analysis of the concept of holism within the context of nursing.' *British Journal of Nursing 2,* 15, 771–775.

Hardy, A. (1979) *The Spiritual Nature of Man: A Study of Contemporary Religious Experience.* Oxford: Clarendon Press.

Hay, D. (1994) 'On the biology of God: what is the current status of Hardy's hypothesis?' *International Journal for the Psychology of Religion 4,* 1, 1–23.

Johnson, D.E. (1980) 'The behavioural systems model for nursing.' In J.P. Riehl and C. Roy (eds) *Conceptual Models for Nursing Practice*, 2nd edn. New York: Appleton-Century-Crofts.

Kenny, T. (1993) 'Nursing models fail in practice.' *British Journal of Nursing 2*, 133–136.

Kolcaba, R. (1997) 'The primary holisms in nursing.' *Journal of Advanced Nursing 25*, 290–296.

Leininger, M.M. (1991) *Cultural Care Diversity and Universality: A Theory of Nursing*. New York: National League for Nursing Press.

Leininger, M.M. (2001) *Culture Care Diversity And Universality: A Theory of Nursing*. Boston: Jones and Bartlett Publishers.

Levine, M.E. (1967) 'The four conservation principles of nursing.' *Nursing Forum 6*, 1, 45–49.

Luker, K. (1988) 'Do models work?' *Nursing Times 88*, 5, 27–28.

Martsolf, D.S. and Mickley, J.R. (1998) 'The concept of spirituality in nursing theories: differing world-views and extent of focus.' *Journal of Advanced Nursing 27*, 294–303.

McSherry, W. (1997) 'A descriptive survey of nurses' perceptions of spirituality and spiritual care.' Unpublished MPhil thesis. Hull: University of Hull.

McSherry, W. (2001) 'Spirituality and learning disabilities: are they compatible?' *Learning Disability Practice 3*, 5, 35–38.

McSherry, W. (2004) 'The meaning of spirituality and spiritual care: an investigation of health care professionals', patients' and public's perceptions.' Unpublished PhD thesis. Leeds: Leeds Metropolitan University.

McSherry, W. and Draper, P. (1998) 'The debates emerging from the literature surrounding the concept of spirituality as applied to nursing.' *Journal of Advanced Nursing 27*, 683–691.

Narayanasamy, A. (1999) 'A review of spirituality as applied to nursing.' *International Journal of Nursing Studies 36*, 117–125.

Neuman, B. (1995) *The Neuman Systems Model*, 3rd edn. Norwalk: Appleton and Lange.

Newberg, A., D'Aquili, E. and Rause, V. (2002) *Why God Won't Go Away: Brain Science and the Biology of Belief*. New York: Ballantine Books.

Newman, M.A. (1986) *Health as Expanding Consciousness*. St Louis: CV Mosby.

Oldnall, A.S. (1995) 'On the absence of spirituality in nursing theories and models.' *Journal of Advanced Nursing 21*, 417–418.

Oldnall, A. (1996) 'A critical analysis of nursing: meeting the spiritual needs of patients.' *Journal of Advanced Nursing 23*, 138–144.

Orem, D.E. (1985) *Nursing: Concepts of Practice*, 3rd edn. New York: McGraw-Hill.

Paley, J. (2002) 'The Cartesian melodrama in nursing.' *Nursing Philosophy 3*, 3, 189–192.

Parse, R.R. (1981) *Man-living-health: A Theory of Nursing*. New York: John Wiley.

Patterson, E.F. (1998) 'The philosophy and physics of holistic health care: spiritual healing as a workable interpretation.' *Journal of Advanced Nursing 27*, 287–293.

Pearson, A., Vaughan, B. and Fitzgerald, M. (2005) *Nursing Models for Practice*, 3rd edn. Oxford: Butterworth Heinemann.

Piles, C. (1990) 'Providing spiritual care.' *Nurse Educator 15*, 1, 36–41.

Rogers, M.E. (1980) 'Nursing: a science of unitary man.' In J.P. Riehl and C. Roy (eds) *Conceptual Models for Nursing Practice*, 2nd edn. New York: Appleton-Century-Crofts.

Roper, N., Logan, W. and Tierney, A. (1980) *The Elements of Nursing: A Model for Nursing Based on a Model of Living*, 2nd edn. Edinburgh: Churchill Livingstone.

Roper, N., Logan, W. and Tierney, A. (1990) *The Elements of Nursing: A Model for Nursing Based on a Model of Living*, 3rd edn. Edinburgh: Churchill Livingstone.

Roy, C. (1980) 'The Roy adaptation model.' In J.P. Riehl and C. Roy (eds) *Conceptual Models for Nursing Practice*, 2nd edn. New York: Appleton-Century-Crofts.

Shelly, J.A. and Fish, S. (1988) *Spiritual Care: The Nurse's Role*, 3rd edn. Illinois: Inter Varsity Press.

Smith, D.W. (1994) 'Toward developing a theory of spirituality.' *Visions 2*, 1, 35–43.

Stallwood, J. and Stoll, R. (1975) 'Spiritual dimensions of nursing practice.' In I.J. Beland and J.Y. Passos (eds) *Clinical Nursing*, 3rd edn. New York: Macmillan.

Stoll, R.I. (1989) 'The essence of spirituality.' In V.B. Carson (ed.) *Spiritual Dimensions of Nursing Practice*. Philadelphia: WB Saunders.

Thorne, S.E. (2001) 'People and their parts: deconstructing the debates in theorizing nursing's clients.' *Nursing Philosophy 2*, 259–262.

Tierney, A.J. (1998) 'Nursing models: extant or extinct?' *Journal of Advanced Nursing 28*, 1, 77–85.

Tournier, P. (1954) *A Doctor's Case Book in the Light of the Bible*. London: SCM Press.

Walsh, M. (1991) *Models in Clinical Nursing – The Way Forward*. London: Baillière Tindall.

Watson, J. (1985) *Nursing: Human Science and Human Care: A Theory of Nursing*. Norwalk: Appleton-Century-Crofts.

Further reading

The concept of holism

These texts will provide you with an insight into the concept of holism. These writings, although written for nursing, have relevance for all health care professionals.

Paley, J. (2002) 'The Cartesian melodrama in nursing.' *Nursing Philosophy 3*, 3, 189–192.

Thorne, S.E. (2001) 'People and their parts: deconstructing the debates in theorizing nursing's clients.' *Nursing Philosophy 2*, 259–262.

Woods, S. (1998) 'Holism in nursing.' In S. Edwards (1998) (ed.) *Philosophical Issues in Nursing*,67–87. London: Macmillan.

Models representing spirituality

By reading the work of these two authors you will gain a deeper understanding of the two models presented in this chapter.

Stallwood, J. and Stoll, R. (1975) 'Spiritual dimensions of nursing practice.' In I.J. Beland and J.Y. Passos (eds) *Clinical Nursing*, 3rd edn. New York: Macmillan.

Stoll, R.I. (1989) 'The essence of spirituality.' In V. Carson (ed.) *Spiritual Dimensions of Nursing Practice.* Philadelphia: WB Saunders.

For an overview of the biological basis of spirituality please read:

Narayanasamy, A. (1999) 'A review of spirituality as applied to nursing.' *International Journal of Nursing Studies 36*, 117–125.

CHAPTER 4

Providing Spiritual Care

Using a Systematic Approach

Introduction

Chapter 2 explored the concept of spirituality, offering several explanations and definitions. These definitions were revisited in Chapter 3 when the concept of spirituality was discussed in relation to holism and conceptual models of care. This chapter covers the concept of spirituality in relation to 'a systematic approach' identifying how spiritual care may be provided within this framework. It is important to remember that individuals who are in need of health care will arrive with their own spirituality and spiritual needs that have developed across their lifespan.

It is wrong to imagine that a person's spirituality, or indeed their spiritual needs, will be left at the entrance of the hospital or outside the care setting. In fact, Murray and Zentner's (1989) definition of spirituality suggests that for some individuals illness or hospitalization may see a refocusing or questioning of their spirituality. An illness, or indeed any crisis, may act as a trigger that moves the individual to revisit, encounter, or 'get in touch with' their own spirituality (Narayanasamy 1996). Therefore, it is not unrealistic to assume that at some point during the course of a health care professional's career they will encounter a patient in their area of practice or under their care who has a spiritual need(s). However, McSherry's (2004) study suggests that not all patients will present with a spiritual need, or even raise any existential or spiritual issues as a result of their illness. Therefore, we cannot make assumptions within health care that all patients or service users will develop or present with spiritual needs(s), or that they will want to discuss matters of a spiritual nature with health care professionals.

Activity 4.1

Before reading the rest of this chapter, spend a few moments reflecting upon your understanding of what is meant by the phrase 'a systematic approach'. Write down any thoughts or experiences that come to mind.

You may well have asked yourself what this exercise has to do with the provision of spiritual care. The answer is that an individual, who is experiencing a spiritual need, as described in Chapter 2, may require such a need to be systematically addressed by the health care professional. Once the need (problem) has been identified, or disclosed by the patient, a goal will need to be formulated. After a prescribed period of time, an evaluation should be undertaken to establish whether the intervention or actions taken by the nurse (team) have been effective. This summary is an oversimplification and there are many issues surrounding spirituality and a systematic approach that will be addressed during the rest of the chapter.

When undertaking Activity 4.1, several thoughts or experiences may have come to mind. First, you may have recalled that a systematic approach is a way of organizing nursing care for patients using a problem-solving approach. Second, you may know that, for example, the nursing process is systematic and cyclical, involving a series of steps or stages starting with assessment and ending with an evaluation of the effectiveness of the care provided (Figure 4.1).

A systematic approach to care, or in nursing the term 'the nursing process', provides a 'safety' mechanism for assessment and evaluation of care. In recent years within nursing (you might want to reflect upon the different innovations within your own profession), numerous types and variations of care plan have come into existence – for example, core care plans (Cowell and Swiers 1997), critical or care pathways (Currie and Harvey 1998) and multidisciplinary collaborative care plans (Scott and Bowen 1997). Despite the emergence of these new methods of recording care, it can be argued that the principles of a systematic approach still apply and are fundamental to their success.

Research undertaken by a host of researchers (see Chapter 7 – Table 7.1) indicates that health care professionals are encountering patients with spiritual needs during the course of their daily practice. Such research findings stress the importance of having some mechanism to ensure that patients' spiritual needs will be effectively addressed and met in health care practice.

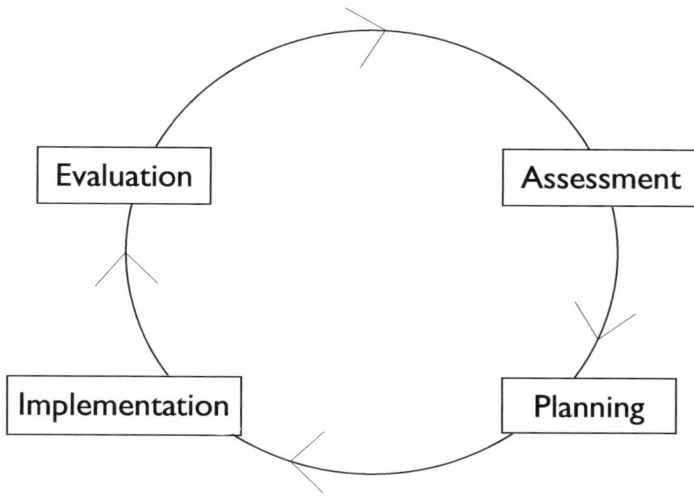

Figure 4.1: Cyclical processes: a systematic approach to care. ***Assessment:*** *Conducting a spiritual assessment, recognizing a patient's spiritual need(s). It is important to be aware that assessment does not end after initial admission but that it is a continuous ongoing process of observation and possible re-assessment.* ***Planning:*** *The identification of those factors that are important to the individual's spirituality. This leads to the setting of goals, short- or long-term, that may be achievable by the individual in meeting his or her spiritual need(s).* ***Implementation:*** *The identification and, where appropriate, the documentation of those interventions that may be instrumental in meeting the spiritual need(s) or enabling the patient to maintain his or her own spiritual needs while ill.* ***Evaluation:*** *The identification of a criterion that may indicate that a patient's spiritual need(s) has been sufficiently addressed. The patient may report a sense of spiritual well-being or a feeling of being at peace with himself or herself or the situation.*

In summary, a systematic approach enables health care professionals to identify a patient's health care problem(s) or needs, placing them in a systematic plan of care that is individualized and patient-centred, irrespective of the patient's underlying condition. The diagram illustrates the cyclical nature of spiritual assessment. We are continuously re-assessing, implementing and re-evaluating care.

A systematic approach to care

Kratz (1979 p.3) states:

> The nursing process is a problem-solving approach to nursing that involves interaction with the patient, making decisions and carrying out nursing actions based on an assessment of an individual patient's situation. It is followed by an evaluation of the effectiveness of our actions.

It is not unreasonable to suspect that this type of systematic approach is familiar to and utilized by many health care professionals in the organization and management of their care. A similar model of systematic assessment is provided by Govier (2000) who proposes that spiritual care can be summarized by the 'Five Rs' (Reason, Reflection, Religion, Relationships and Restoration) and delivered within a cyclical process, while Whipp (2001), when discussing the application of theological audit in health care organizations, presents an audit model that may lead to improvement in operational aspects of patient care. Therefore, it is not unreasonable or unrealistic to apply this systematic approach to an individual who presents with a spiritual need, nor is it unrealistic to suggest that the majority of health care professionals would feel comfortable and familiar with this form of care delivery. Ross (1996) suggests that spiritual care should be delivered to patients and taught to nurses, and this recommendation could be extended to include all health professions within the framework of the nursing process or a systematic approach. However, in recent times, the nursing process or a systematic approach has been the subject of much debate and criticism. Marks-Maran (1999) feels that it is now outdated.

Despite recent criticism, the four stages involved in the systematic approach – assessment, planning, implementation and evaluation (Figure 4.1) – can still be applied to problems of a spiritual nature (Harrison and Burnard 1993). Each of these stages will be addressed in detail during the rest of the chapter. However, it must be emphasized that the main principles of a systematic approach may need to be modified to meet an individual's circumstances. Spiritual problems do not fit neatly into each stage of the cyclical process because these needs are usually complex. In fact, spiritual needs may go unrecognized during an initial assessment (McSherry 1996). These issues will be explored through the use of case studies and reflective exercises.

Documentation

Another point that must be borne in mind when introducing a systematic approach is the issue of documentation. The importance of documentation or record-keeping within health care has generated much debate in relation to legal and ethical issues and who might have access to such information (Data Protection Act 1998). You are also encouraged to look at the implications of the Caldicott Report (DH 1997) which has led to the publications and guidance for NHS staff and, more recently, for people working in social care when dealing with issues of confidentiality and patient information (DH 2003). In stressing the importance of documentation, a simple principle applies. If a nurse's, or indeed any health care professional's, care or actions are disputed, bringing into question the quality or standard of the care provided, then if nothing is written there will be nothing in their defence – a 'belt and braces mentality'. However, where a patient's or service user's problem originates from the spiritual dimension, owing to the sensitive and deeply personal nature of the issue identified, it may not be appropriate to document the concern or even devise a care plan. Patient confidentiality and consent is a very important issue when providing spiritual care. These legal and ethical issues will be addressed towards the end of the chapter.

Assessment

The first stage in a systematic approach is assessment of an individual's care needs. Assessment involves the gathering of information, perhaps from a wide range of sources – i.e. patient, medical records or family – by various means such as questioning or observation, in order to identify the patient's actual or potential problems. As you may recall, an assessment framework that is widely used in the UK involves the twelve activities of daily living based on or derived from the Roper, Logan and Tierney 'model of living' (1990), and this type of model or a similar one is used by many health care professionals. These activities are used as a checklist or template to provide some structure for the initial or admission assessment depending upon whether the context of care is primary, secondary or tertiary.

Activity 4.2

Read Case study 4.1. Then write down on a piece of paper the types of questions that you might ask Mr Smith during the admission procedure.

Case study 4.1 Looking beyond the obvious

Mr Smith, a 75-year-old retired miner, is admitted onto your ward or under your care with a chest infection. Mr Smith has been unwell for several weeks. He has become extremely breathless upon exertion and has developed a productive cough. He reports that he has recently been bereaved, his wife dying from breast cancer.

The admitting nurse or health care professional might use the twelve activities of daily living as a mechanism for systematically enquiring into all aspects of the individual's life – in principle, an individualized, patient-centred and holistic approach, providing a comprehensive and detailed assessment of the individual's normal function and subsequent needs (Table 4.1). However, the assessment and identification of a patient's spiritual needs may be problematic. Because of the sensitive nature of spirituality, an individual may not share or reveal such information during an initial assessment since spirituality is normally incorporated under the section 'dying'. However, many care plans or admission records now incorporate a section entitled 'spiritual needs'. With regards to spiritual assessment, a number of frameworks or assessment tools have been developed that may assist health care professionals in exploring the spiritual dimension of their patients or service users (Box 4.1).

Undertaking this exercise may have been easy in relation to several of the categories that address physical activities, such as eating, drinking or breathing. Similarly, we may feel comfortable with asking specific questions relating to our professional role – for example, a physiotherapist may enquire into the impact of the breathlessness upon mobility while a dietician may focus upon appetite, and the occupational therapist may explore personal activities such as washing and dressing. However, there may have been some areas of Mr Smith's life that were difficult to assess – for example, his recent bereavement, his own attitudes towards death and dying, or even issues surrounding spiritual needs or sexuality. It has been recognized that there are several aspects of health care that are considered taboo; these include sexuality, death and dying, and matters concerning spirituality. Nurses and other health care practitioners may overlook these areas when assessing a patient (Burnard 1988).

Table 4.1 Admission assessment based on the activities of daily living

Normal activity of daily living	Changes due to present illness/admission	Problem no.	Signature and date
Maintaining a safe Environment			
Eating and drinking			
Breathing: Mr Smith smokes 30 cigarettes per day. He has no family history of breathing problems such as asthma or bronchitis.	Mr Smith reports that he has become very breathless upon the slightest of exertion. He has noticed a wheeze and says that he is coughing up thick green sputum.		
Elimination			
Communication			
Washing and dressing			
Mobilizing			
Temperature			
Dying	Mr Smith reports that he has recently been bereaved, and his wife died of breast cancer six months ago. He states that he has no fears about death and that 'when you are dead, that's the end of everything.'		
Sleeping			
Working and recreation: Mr Smith worked as a miner for 35 years before being made redundant after the mines closed. He likes to have a game of darts, a couple of nights a week, at his local with his mates.	Mr Smith feels that he will miss his weekly visits to his local for a pint and a game of darts – 'Since my wife's death I like the company.'		

Table 4.1 *cont.*

Normal activity of daily living	Changes due to present illness/admission	Problem no.	Signature and date
Expressing sexuality:			
Spiritual needs: Mr Smith devoted a great deal of time caring for his wife who had terminal cancer. He does not believe in any life after death. He is adamant that there is no God and that religion is only trouble.	Mr Smith feels that since becoming ill he has started to question what life is all about. He finds it difficult to understand why some individuals seem to have more suffering and pain than others. He states that he does not want to see a chaplain.		

Box 4.1 Summary of published frameworks/models used in the advancement of spiritual issues

Highfield (1993)
Acronym PLAN
P: Permission
L: Limited information
A: Activating resources
N: Non-nursing assistance

Govier (2000)
Five 'R's of spirituality:
Reasons
Reflection
Religion
Relationships
Restoration

Ross (1996)
McSherry (2000)
A systematic cyclical approach, incorporating the five phases:

Assessment
Planning
Implementation
Evaluation, and reassessment

Narayanasamy (1999, 2001)

ASSET Model (Actioning spirituality and spiritual care education and training in nursing)

ACCESS
A: Assessment
C: Communication
C: Cultural negotiation and compromise
E: Establishing respect and rapport
S: Sensitivity
S: Safety

Puchalski and Romer (2000)

Acronym FICA
F: Faith or beliefs
I: Importance and influence
C: Community
A: Address

Anandarajah and Hight (2001)

Acronym HOPE
H: sources of hope, meaning, comfort, strength, peace, love and connection
O: Organized religion
P: Personal spirituality and practices
E: Effects on medical care and end-of-life issues

Source: Nyatanga and Astley-Pepper (2005, p.115)

Activity 4.3

Reflecting upon your own clinical experience, can you recall the number of care plans you have encountered that have addressed or identified in detail a patient's spirituality or spiritual needs?

Your reflections may reveal that you have encountered very few care plans or admission assessment forms that have identified a patient's spiritual need(s) while in hospital or out in the community. You may have recalled that in the 'spiritual needs' section the patient's religious beliefs had been written as C of E (Church of England) or RC (Roman Catholic). You may also have identified that on many occasions the section was left blank or empty. There are several reasons for the box remaining blank; these are listed in Box 4.2.

Box 4.2 Reasons for spiritual needs section being left empty

The subject of spiritual needs is too intrusive and personal to address on admission.

The admitting health care professional nurse did not feel comfortable in addressing such questions.

The patient did not want to answer the question or did not identify any spiritual needs at the time of admission.

The patient, and indeed the nurse, did not understand the term 'spiritual needs'.

The patient identified a spiritual need considered too private and sensitive to write or disclose in his or her care plan.

In order to address the fears and apprehensions that health care professionals may experience when asked to address or assess matters of a spiritual nature, several authors have devised questions or guidelines that may make spiritual assessment easier.

Stoll (1979) presents some guidelines for undertaking a spiritual assessment:

> *Concept of God or deity.* The types of questions that may be asked by the nurse addressing this aspect of spirituality are: Is religion or God significant to you? If yes, can you describe how? Is prayer helpful to you? What happens when you pray? (p.1572)
>
> *Sources of hope and strength.* Who is the most important person to you? To whom do you turn when you need help? Are they available? (p.1575)

Religious practices. Do you feel that your faith (or religion) is helpful to you? If yes, would you tell me how? Are there any religious practices that are important to you? (p.1576)

Relationship between spiritual beliefs and health. What has bothered you most about being sick (or in what is happening to you)? What do you think is going to happen to you? (pp.1576–1577)

Activity 4.4

Spend several minutes reflecting upon these guidelines and write down your first impressions.

It is suggested that assessment in relation to the identification of spiritual needs must be an 'ongoing' exercise. Questioning an individual about his or her religious orientation or spiritual needs may be appropriate and helpful on admission to hospital, or when first meeting them in the community, in identifying those individuals for whom religious affiliation and practice are fundamental to their spiritual well-being. However, caution must be exercised as for the unbeliever, atheist or agnostic (Burnard 1988) this type of questioning may be threatening. Stoll's guidelines do suggest the types of areas that may need to be addressed within a spiritual assessment. She herself, towards the end of her article (Stoll 1979, p.1577), writes:

> Neither sexual nor spiritual values should be introduced at the beginning of the interview. I have found it beneficial to separate sexuality from spiritual concerns with questions pertaining to physical and social needs. The spiritual dimension lends itself to being a continuation of the psychosocial assessment toward the latter part of an interview.

This quotation highlights the sensitivity that has to be employed when discussing spiritual concerns. Two major questions must be considered before nurses, chaplains and academics 'steam roll' ahead in designing complex assessment criteria:

1. Can spiritual needs be identified by the use of assessment tools – for example, those used to predict or identify those individuals at risk of developing a pressure sore, i.e. Waterlow score? Or using

visual analogue scales to identify the amount and type of spiritual pain an individual may be experiencing?

2. Can spiritual needs be predicted by such mechanistic interventions and calculations? The definitions of spirituality presented in Chapter 2 demonstrate that it is a very subjective, complex and individually determined aspect of life.

CAUTION

There is a danger in making spiritual assessment mechanistic, reducing it to a tick box exercise that may negate the use of other modes of continuous assessment (Catterall *et al.* 1998). This can be illustrated by the following question: What if a patient is assessed on admission by one nurse or health care professional who, at that time, felt the patient did not have any spiritual needs? Does this mean that such an individual may not develop a spiritual need(s) during the course of their illness or hospitalization? If you can recall Murray and Zentner's (1989) definition, this seems to support the principle of continuous assessment because during their period of illness or hospitalization individuals may begin to question the meaning of life or the implications of illness (Simsen 1985), perhaps facing the prospect of death. Such existential questions may not be raised, or identified, when a patient is first admitted into hospital. The dangers or problems that can arise when even the crudest of spiritual assessments is not undertaken during admission to hospital are raised in Case study 4.2.

Case study 4.2 Spiritual care: a case to answer

Peter, 72 years old, was known by his family and friends to like a short or two. He was admitted to hospital with an acute episode of chest pain. A diagnosis of angina was made since ECGs showed no evidence of recent infarct.

It came to light later that Peter was a practising Roman Catholic who found meaning and purpose in his beliefs. Peter had only been in hospital overnight and he had not seen his wife because she had taken herself off to their daughters 'down south' after an argument. Nevertheless, she was informed by Peter of his admission into hospital and she was intending to visit as soon as possible. In the afternoon on the following day Peter was due to be discharged when he developed sudden severe central chest pain, collapsing with a cardiac arrest – resuscitation was initiated. During the resuscitation, Peter's wife arrived on the ward. Unfortunately, she did not see Peter before he died. After Peter's death, his wife asked if the Catholic priest had been. Inspection of the nursing notes showed that nothing in relation to religion had been entered.

Activity 4.5

Having read the case study surrounding Peter, can you identify any issues that you feel it generates in relation to the assessment of an individual's spiritual needs?

In response to this question, you may have identified that there is an important need for a brief assessment of an individual's religious orientation and practices. In Peter's case, his religious beliefs were a fundamental part of his spirituality. His Catholic faith had become interwoven into his beliefs and all dimensions of his life. By omitting to identify Peter's religious practices, the nurses had failed in their duty to provide 'holistic' care. The case study stresses the role of the nurse in documenting even the simplest of information. We are all probably guilty of skipping the question surrounding religion, as demonstrated when reflecting upon your own practice earlier. Peter's case highlights the important role that nurses play in communicating, maintaining and identifying a patient's religious practices to others in the multidisciplinary team such as the hospital chaplains or the patient's own religious leader. A failure to undertake the crudest of spiritual assessments, which may initially only ask about a patient's religious beliefs and practices, can prove detrimental to the patient. It could be argued that Peter's case is extreme, but nevertheless it highlights the important point that there is no room for complacency when addressing matters of spirituality.

The case study demonstrates how failure to provide spiritual care may influence the attitudes of patients and their next of kin about the standard and quality of care being provided. One cannot read Peter's case without thinking that the nursing profession had failed Peter and his wife. She had witnessed care that was fragmented and not individual because it was ineffectual in that it did not recognize her husband's spirituality.

It has been suggested in this section that assessment of spiritual needs should be ongoing and continuous. There are several methods or measures that can be used that assist in identifying a patient who has a spiritual need(s) (adapted from Carson 1989, p.158):

> *Direct questioning.* We have demonstrated that this may be inappropriate, threatening and perceived as intrusive. However, it may be used to elicit information quickly about religious beliefs and practices upon admission.
>
> *Observation of non-verbal and verbal behaviour.* The individual may be withdrawn or look and act frustrated or agitated. His or her body language may suggest that the person is depressed. The person may physically seek solitude or isolation (McSherry 1996). Does the person pray or use other symbolic gestures? However, it must be stressed that these types of behaviour may also be indicative of concern that is not related to a spiritual need but still requires addressing. With reference to the verbal behaviours that may indicate that a person has a spiritual need, you may notice that the individual is always complaining out of all proportion. He or she may call upon God in a derogatory way. During the course of a conversation the patient may question the meaning of his or her health problem, life or future prognosis. These forms of verbal behaviour may indicate that an individual is having difficulty accepting or reconciling some issue that is affecting his or her very existence, or they may be indicative of an issue that is nothing to do with the person's spirituality.
>
> *Interpersonal.* Most patients have visitors or family and friends. However, there may be occasions when a patient does not have anyone visiting. This may indicate that a person is living alone and perhaps is isolated – a point worth clarifying with the person. Some patients may have representatives of their faith visiting frequently, indicating their belief and involvement in a particular faith. On odd occasions after a patient has had visitors, he or she may appear frustrated, angered or annoyed, indicating that their relationships are not entirely harmonious or supportive.
>
> *Environmental.* The patient might wear a religious artefact, such as a medal or a cross. Their cards may be of a religious nature. They may read religious

material or holy books such as the Bible. The example in Case study 4.3 illustrates the importance of observational assessment.

Case study 4.3 Importance of environmental cues

An elderly man had been admitted onto the ward several days earlier for medical observation and assessment for bowel problems. In the night he required an emergency operation. When gathering together the patient's belongings to transfer them across to the surgical ward while the patient was in theatre, nurses came across an old Bible with dog-eared pages. This revealed the patient's personal belief in a God. It also alerted nurses to the fact that the man did have a personal spiritual belief that nurses could help him meet. The man had been too ill to disclose his beliefs on admission and he had no family or friends for anyone to ask.

Elizabeth Johnston Taylor (2002, pp.103–136) provides her readers with a useful summary of the vast array of models for spiritual assessment. However, before health care professionals rush off and start to utilize such models, consideration must be given to some of the dilemmas that surround this area of health care practice (Johnson 2001; McSherry and Ross 2002).

Planning

After assessment, there is a need to use the information gained to formulate a plan of care. Where possible this should be done in collaboration with the patient/service user. The information should be collated and verified with the patient and then goal(s) should be set that are realistic, patient-centred and in a time frame that is acceptable to the patient and the health care professional. Planning is probably the most difficult aspect of using a problem-solving or systematic approach. With reference to a physical problem such as nausea and vomiting, or relieving the discomfort associated with a high temperature, the plan or goal can usually be drawn up easily. For example, Mrs Jones will report that her nausea has been relieved within 30 minutes of it developing. The formulation of such goals is not so easy with problems arising from a spiritual need(s).

Activity 4.6

Re-read Case study 2.2 and the subsequent section addressing Jim's spiritual needs (the case study is reproduced here as Case study 4.4). Now devise a plan of care that you feel would enable Jim to meet the spiritual need shown by his loss of meaning, purpose and fulfilment.

Case study 4.4 Time to think

Jim, 65 years old, was admitted to the ward with a grossly swollen right leg, thigh and calf. A diagnosis of DVT (deep vein thrombosis) was made. He was started on a heparin infusion and kept on total bed rest because of the severe pain when he mobilized.

One morning, while the nurse was talking to Jim, he became very emotional and began to cry. As the nurse listened to him, it emerged that on 24 December it was the first anniversary of his wife's death. Jim recalled how he had been married for 45 years and for the last 10 years of his married life had been the main carer for his wife, who suffered from rheumatoid arthritis. Jim went on to describe how lonely and depressed he felt, stating that a day did not pass without him thinking about his wife and the wonderful life they had shared together. Jim was not a religious man but he did believe in life after death.

Having read the case study, you have probably identified that Jim has several different spiritual needs that need to be addressed, such as the need for meaning and purpose, the need for trust and a need for a loving relationship. You may also have found it difficult to articulate or write a goal. The overall result may be one of frustration, leaving only a series of questions:

- How do you go about setting goals and establishing a criterion against which spiritual needs can be measured?
- How do you determine whether a goal can be met in the short or long term?

- Are there not some ethical issues about writing down something that is deeply personal and private?
- How can you write a goal for needs that seem so subjective and complex?

The writing and formulation of care plans is often very difficult and time-consuming. It could be argued that one reason for having core care plans or critical pathways is to reduce the amount of time that qualified nurses spend on completing paperwork. Time spent with paperwork could mean less time spent with the patient. However, such sentiments would not stand up in a court of law – remember, if there is nothing written, then there is nothing in your defence. Core care plans or critical pathways do not really accommodate the subjective and complex nature of spiritual needs because such needs are so unique and individually determined that they do not lend themselves to flow charts or tick box exercises. Therefore, if a patient's or service user's spiritual needs are to be addressed in a plan of care, then usually the nurse or health care professional will have to work through each stage in a systematic approach. A goal needs to be formulated and time limits for evaluation set, with the planning taking place in conjunction with the patient.

Goals

Setting goals that can address spiritual needs requires flexibility and sensitivity. Goals should be grounded in reality – they should be achievable. A problem with some spiritual needs is that they cannot be resolved in the short term. For example, in Case study 4.4, Jim had lost meaning and purpose in his life after the death of his wife. It would be totally unrealistic to expect the goals for his spiritual care to be met overnight (see Box 4.3). There are many issues that Jim will have to face and explore before his life has new meaning and purpose. It is the lack of concrete solutions and quick fixes that makes the setting of goals difficult when trying to address a patient's spiritual need(s). It is very likely that it will take Jim many months before he has totally come to terms with the death of his wife and resolved the loss and spiritual pain that he experienced. Having stated this, it is not unrealistic to start a patient on the journey of reflection and acceptance while in hospital or under the care of a health professional.

Box 4.3 Jim's plan of care

Identified patient concern/problem

Jim has identified that he has lost all meaning and purpose in life, and that he feels lonely and depressed since his wife's death.

Goal

While in hospital, the goal is to enable Jim to evaluate his life in order to rediscover value, meaning and purpose.

Plan of care

The health care professional should allow time for Jim to explore and discuss the fears and worries that have destroyed meaning and value in his life.

All members of staff should treat Jim with dignity and respect, fostering a relationship of trust – perhaps restoring confidence and hope.

The health care professional should identify with Jim the areas in his life that he may find enjoyable and meaningful, using these as a platform on which to build self-esteem.

If it was felt appropriate, Jim could refer himself to an external agency that would be able to provide support and counselling upon discharge.

Implementation

Implementing a plan of care means that energy and time are being committed to reaching a desired goal or outcome that has been set by the patient or service user in conjunction with the health care professional. With reference to the meeting of a spiritual need, the plan usually involves an element of time on the health care professional's part spent actively listening to the patient's concerns. Time may also be spent liaising with others in the multidisciplinary team – for example, informing or arranging a visit by the hospital chaplain or the patient's or service user's own religious or spiritual leader. The plan of care may also see the health care professional organizing the environment in order to allow the individual time alone and privacy in which to pray or reflect. The plan of care will ultimately be determined by whatever spiritual need(s) a patient or service user presents with. A patient or service user whose spiritual need(s) are based on maintaining their spiritual practices may be accommodated by allowing time for them to pray or read in private. It may entail organizing care and staff so that the patient or service user can attend a communion service in the chapel on Sunday or a holy day of obligation. It may also involve staff being sensitive and respectful of individuals who are following certain religious festivals or fasts. It may mean contacting the patient's religious or spiritual leaders and notifying them that they have been admitted into hospital or that an individual has died so that specific rites and rituals can be performed in accordance with the person's religious customs. This reinforces the need to obtain as much detail and information about a person's religious practices upon admission so that insight can be gained and appropriate actions implemented.

The critical incident analysis in Case study 4.5 demonstrates how detailed assessment influences all the different stages in the nursing process – planning, implementation, right through to evaluation. Effective spiritual care cannot be offered to a patient or service user unless sufficient information has been obtained during assessment (continuous) and communicated to all staff involved in care delivery – from consultant to housekeeper. A plan of care that highlights what an individual's spiritual need(s) are and how these needs are to be met allows everyone to work together to achieve the desired goal. Spiritual care, indeed all types of care, will be fragmented and goals will not be effectively reached if everyone is working in isolation and implementing their own plan of care. You may recall how frustrating it can be when you have applied a particular wound dressing for a patient, or written specific instructions in the care plan for certain dietary supplements to be given, only to find, on your return, that one of your colleagues has ignored your plan of care and applied something different from what you documented or not given any of the recommended dietary supplements. Continuity is lost and everyone, including the patient service user, is left feeling confused. This illustration also highlights issues of accountability.

Case study 4.5 Critical incident analysis

A patient had not really eaten a substantial meal since being admitted into hospital two days previously. The patient in question had suffered a stroke several years earlier that had left him with expression dysphasia. Investigating the matter, it emerged that the patient was a vegan and since admission had been given meat or dairy products at meal times. With insight, it was obvious why the patient had refused to eat, as he had been offended by the diet offered. This critical incident analysis highlights the value and importance individuals attach to their own personal, cultural beliefs and practices. It also reinforces the need for a systematic way of communicating and implementing patient care.

Evaluation

Evaluation is the final stage in using a systematic approach to care, and possibly the most difficult to undertake in relation to establishing whether an individual's spiritual need(s) have been met. Health care interventions that seek to address physical problems are usually easier to review. For example, making tracings or taking photographs of a patient's leg ulcer upon admission or before commencing a treatment regime would provide a baseline for subsequent evaluation. Three weeks later, the ulcer is retraced or new photographs taken. Comparisons with the drawings or photographs will reveal any improvement or deterioration, indicating whether the care is effective or the desired goal achieved.

The same principle can be applied to an individual whose spiritual needs have their origin within a religious framework. It is easy to establish whether these types of spiritual need have been met by ensuring the patient attends a particular service or documenting that their religious/spiritual leader has been to visit. However, things are not so 'black and white' when trying to evaluate spiritual needs that are very subjective, involving the ordinary and mundane aspects of life. As you will recall, spiritual needs are uniquely determined by the individual. The problems arise because there is no baseline or criterion against which future comparisons can be made and progress determined. For example, how does the health care professional set about reviewing or evaluating whether a person is starting to regain meaning and purpose in life? Or how does one determine whether a person feels reconciled or forgiven? These two questions indicate the problematic nature of evaluating whether a patient's or service user's spiritual needs have been met.

Consultation and participation are the two key ingredients in determining the effectiveness of spiritual interventions. The patient or service user should be consulted and asked to comment upon how he or she feels that progress is being made towards meeting a specific spiritual need. The patient or service user might reveal that he or she is feeling more optimistic about the future.

Another indicator that a spiritual need is being addressed may be found in how an individual describes himself or herself. Words like relaxed, at peace, or inner calm may indicate a refocusing of spirituality. Earlier the importance of observation as a means of assessment was discussed. As with assessment, observation can be used as an aid to evaluation. The nurse may observe verbal and non-verbal behaviours that may indicate a change in attitude or inner disposition. An individual who was extremely withdrawn may display behaviour that suggests a more relaxed openness towards staff or other patients – communicating more freely.

Difficulties

Another problem with evaluation is the setting of realistic time limits for review. As stated earlier, it may take an individual many months to come to terms with a health problem or personal crisis that has brought into question his or her entire existence. It would be unrealistic to expect such an individual to reflect, adjust and regain composure in a matter of hours, days or possibly weeks. Therefore, setting realistic dates for the review of a spiritual need must take into consideration the individual and the spiritual need that has been identified or disclosed. To say that it will take three days for a patient to establish trust and one week for an individual to regain meaning and purpose in his or her life after a diagnosis of Type II diabetes mellitus would be very prescriptive. This type of approach would be totally unrealistic and ineffective, contradicting everything that has been discussed in this chapter. Therefore, evaluation of spiritual needs requires sensitivity and common sense in that there needs to be a realization on the nurse's part that individuals will meet their own spiritual needs at a pace determined by the patients themselves.

This section has highlighted the difficulties associated with evaluation of spiritual needs, especially those needs that are very subjective. Having stated this, evaluation needs to be undertaken in order to assess an individual's progress, and to identify any measures that the nurse can implement to assist in the goal being met. If problems are encountered, then the goal may need to be re-assessed and an alternative strategy devised and implemented.

Ethical considerations

Throughout this chapter, you may be pausing and reflecting upon the material, asking yourself several fundamental questions around assessment, documentation, continuity of care, accountability and confidentiality.

Activity 4.7

Read Case study 4.6 and identify any ethical issues that you feel are apparent or applicable to this case.

Case study 4.6 is complex, addressing several important aspects of spirituality such as the need for inner peace (McSherry 1996). The case study reinforces how spirituality is related to all aspects of a person's being. Reading the case study, you may identify several important ethical issues raised, such as confidentiality, accountability and advocacy. These ethical issues bring into question many of the principles surrounding the use of the nursing process or documentation as a framework for providing spiritual care.

Case study 4.6 The need for a team approach

Pamela, 27 years old, was admitted to the ward with a recent history of weight loss and anorexia. On admission, she looked very pale and thin and had a body mass index of 19, indicating that she was possibly malnourished. The medical team could find no physical or pathological explanation to account for her condition.

Pamela was a highly anxious individual who had been suffering from anxiety and depression for several months. Therefore, the medical team concluded that her anorexia and weight loss were associated with her high anxiety state. She was seen by a dietician and referred to a psychiatrist.

Pamela had a great deal of support and understanding from her partner, with whom she had three children. During the course of her hospitalization, she became very emotional and frustrated at the medical staff's inability to find any physical explanation for her condition. On one occasion, she ran off following a procedure that did not discover any pathology and was found sitting outside, crying bitterly. After being encouraged and supported back to the day room, Pamela revealed to the nurse that she had had a termination of pregnancy earlier that year, which she now felt ashamed and embarrassed about. She recalled how at that time her partner was out of work, having been made redundant, and they felt that financially it would be unfair to bring another child into their family.

Owing to numerous interruptions in the day room, the nurse felt that it would be unfair to continue with the conversation and that they should resume it at another time. Pamela did state that she had always been an anxious individual, but her anxiety and depression had increased soon after this event; she asked the nurse not to mention this to anyone. The following day, the nurse arrived back on duty to find that Pamela had been discharged home that morning with an outpatient appointment to see the psychiatrist and dietician.

Continuity of care

In the case study, the nurse was starting to address a spiritual need, only to find that the patient had been discharged. Pamela's situation highlights the difficulties that patients and health care professionals may encounter when disclosing and addressing spiritual concerns. The circumstances in the case study reveal how continuity of care can be problematic. This raises a question: How ethical is it to start to address a patient's spiritual pain – possibly 'opening a can of worms' – to find that there is no means of closure or developing a relationship that may be therapeutic? The fast throughput of patients in acute and critical care settings may mean that the continuity of care that is vital if patients' and service users' spiritual needs are to be effectively met can be limited. Pamela's case underlines the need for a team approach in the meeting of patients' spiritual needs. It is no good just the nurses being spiritually aware. This awareness and sensitivity towards problems of a spiritual nature needs to be adopted by medical and other professions allied to medicine. If this awareness is not universally shared, then spiritual needs in patients will always go unrecognized or dismissed as undeserving of medical attention or intervention. In some instances, a referral to the psychiatrist or hospital chaplain may be counter-productive.

Discharge policy

Another important issue in relation to continuity is discharge planning and referrals. It has been indicated that spiritual needs that are complex, involving matters addressing meaning, purpose and fulfilment in life, may not be resolved in the short term. Is it ethical and reasonable to expect nurses or chaplains to provide support to individuals with such needs while in hospital, if they are to be discharged with the individual's spiritual concerns only partially addressed? This point brings into question issues about continuity of care between acute and community, primary care settings. Interestingly, the National Health Service Executive (Northern and Yorkshire regions) in 1995 devised 'a framework for spiritual faith and pastoral related care' (Institute of Nursing 1995). Close inspection of this document does not give any acknowledgement to this problem. Neither does the framework make any suggestions as to how solutions to this ethical dilemma may be formulated. It would appear that there is an urgent need to develop a national standard that addresses these problems of continuity of care. Recent developments in the provision of spiritual care have seen organisations produce strategy documents – for example, South Yorkshire NHS Workforce Development Confederation (2003) produced 'Caring for the spirit: a strategy for the chaplaincy and spiritual healthcare workforce'. These strategic approaches may ensure continuity of care amongst all sectors.

Documentation (revisited)

Throughout this chapter, the importance of documentation has been emphasized. However, Pamela's case study demonstrates the personal and sensitive nature of spiritual needs. Would it have been right to have written something so personal and confidential in a plan of care, with the potential for everyone to read it? Another area of concern would be if Pamela had asked specifically for all the information she had entrusted to the nurse to remain private and confidential – neither wanting anything written nor anything verbally disclosed. This type of request can be very challenging and threatening because the nurse is torn 'between the devil and the deep blue sea'. The dilemma is that, if you do not disclose or document something, then an event may occur that could have been prevented if others had been fully informed. However, there are no easy ethical solutions and the result is often to be found in collaboration and communication within a safe and confidential relationship between the patient and the nurse in whom the patient has confided.

Confidentiality

Pamela's case study highlights the deeply personal and sensitive nature of spirituality. It demonstrates clearly how situations and circumstances in life can change, bringing into question motives and moral decision-making and reasoning. However, would it have been right for the nurse to have disclosed such personal facts to other staff? Should such personal situations be documented in a plan of care? These are very important questions that nurses must ask when addressing matters of a spiritual nature. Patients may feel more secure if they know that a problem they have divulged to you is safe. You are probably well aware that any breach of confidentiality, however small, can destroy the patient's trust, and all measures being taken to help meet a patient's spiritual needs will be futile. Such dilemmas put the nurse in a very precarious situation, a little like the priest in a confessional who receives some information that could save lives but where the details cannot be disclosed because of the seal of confession. To say that there are easy solutions to such dilemmas would be very prescriptive and unrealistic. Many of these situations are dependent upon individual circumstances and usually solutions are to be found in the situation itself. An example of this is that often after some time reflecting, the patient may acknowledge that there is a need for further help and ask for the information to be passed on to the appropriate professionals or agencies. However, this does not remove or diminish the level of responsibility or pressure that a nurse may experience when he or she is privy to confidential matters concerning a patient. At times, being responsible for such information can leave individual nurses feeling under pressure and both emotionally challenged and isolated.

Advocacy

This implies that health care professionals should act in a manner that will promote and safeguard the interests and well-being of patients or clients within the sphere of their care. The principle of advocacy is often difficult and problematic to apply in practice. This is evident in Pamela's situation. In order to address Pamela's spiritual needs, and maintain trust and confidence, the nurse is obliged not to disclose the spiritual matters that have resulted in her loss of spiritual well-being. On the other hand, the nurse is aware that, if the spiritual needs are documented and disclosed, then this will inform the course of her care and subsequent decisions made by the medical and nursing team.

Conclusion

This chapter has explored how spiritual care can be provided within a systematic framework involving assessment, planning, implementation and evaluation. Through the use of case studies, spiritual needs that may arise within clinical practice have been presented. Implicitly, it is acknowledged that the entire area of care planning, case management and documentation are fundamental in the delivery of the highest quality health care. This principle is also relevant when addressing patients or service users whose problems have their origin within the spiritual realm. The information provided addressing spirituality and a systematic approach is not prescriptive, acknowledging that there are no easy solutions to be found to often complex ethical dilemmas. The chapter has emphasized the need for reflection upon practice in order to develop insight and new knowledge.

References

Anandarajah, G. and Hight, E. (2001) 'Spirituality and medical practice: using the HOPE questions as a practical tool for spiritual assessment.' *American Family Physician 63*, 1, 81–88.

Burnard, P. (1988) 'The spiritual needs of atheists and agnostics.' *Professional Nurse* December: 130–132.

Carson, V.B. (1989) *Spiritual Dimensions of Nursing Practice.* Philadelphia: WB Saunders.

Catterall, R.A., Cox, M., Greet, B., Sankey, J. and Griffiths, G. (1998) 'The assessment and audit of spiritual care.' *International Journal of Palliative Nursing 4*, 4, 162–168.

Cowell, J. and Swiers, D. (1997) 'Trust-wide core care plans.' *Nursing Standard 12*, 4, 39–41.

Currie, L. and Harvey, G. (1998) 'Care pathways development and implementation.' *Nursing Standard 12*, 30, 35–38.

Data Protection Act 1998. Available from: www.opsi.gov.uk/acts/acts1998/199980020.htm

Department of Health (DH) (1997) *The Caldicott Committee Report on the Review of Patient-Identifiable Information.* London: DH.

Department of Health (2003) *Confidentiality NHS Code of Practice.* London: DH.

Govier, I. (2000) 'Spiritual care in nursing: a systematic approach.' *Nursing Standard 14*, 17, 32–36.

Harrison, J. and Burnard, P. (1993) *Spirituality and Nursing Practice.* Aldershot: Avebury.

Highfield, M.E. (1993) 'PLAN: a spiritual care model for every nurse.' *Quality of Life – A Nursing Challenge 2*, 3, 80–84.

Institute of Nursing (1995) *A Framework for Spiritual, Faith and Related Pastoral Care.* Leeds: Institute of Nursing, University of Leeds.

Johnson, C.P. (2001) 'Assessment tools: are they an effective approach to implementing spiritual health care within the NHS?' *Accident and Emergency Nursing 9*, 177–186.

Kratz, C.R. (1979) *The Nursing Process.* London: Baillière Tindall.

Marks-Maran, D. (1999) 'Reconstructing nursing: evidence, artistry and curriculum.' *Nurse Education Today 19*, 3–10.

McSherry, W. (1996) 'Raising the spirits.' *Nursing Times 92*, 3, 48–49.

McSherry, W. (2000) *Making Sense of Spirituality in Nursing Practice: An Interactive Approach.* Edinburgh: Churchill Livingstone.

McSherry, W. (2004) 'The meaning of spirituality and spiritual care: an investigation of health care professionals', patients' and public's perceptions.' Unpublished PhD thesis. Leeds: Leeds Metropolitan University.

McSherry, W. (2005) 'Spirituality and Palliative Care' in Nyatanga, B., and Astley-Pepper, M. (2005) *Hidden Aspects of Palliative Care.* London: Quay Books.

McSherry, W. and Ross, L. (2002) 'Dilemmas of spiritual assessment: considerations for nursing practice.' *Journal of Advanced Nursing 38*, 5, 479–488.

Murray, R.B. and Zentner, J.B. (1989) *Nursing Concepts for Health Promotion.* London: Prentice Hall.

Narayanasamy, A. (1996) 'Spiritual care of chronically ill patients.' *British Journal of Nursing 5*, 7, 411–416.

Narayanasamy, A. (1999) 'ASSET: a model for actioning spirituality and spiritual care education and training in nursing.' *Nurse Education Today 19*, 274–285.

Narayanasamy, A. (2001) *Spiritual Care: A Practical Guide for Nurses and Health Care Practitioners*, 2nd edn. Wiltshire: Quay Publishing.

Puchalski, C. and Romer, A.L. (2000) 'Taking a spiritual history allows clinicians to understand patients more fully.' *Journal of Palliative Medicine 3*, 1, 129–137.

Roper, N., Logan, W. and Tierney, A. (1990) *The Elements of Nursing: A Model for Nursing Based on a Model of Living*, 3rd edn. Edinburgh: Churchill Livingstone.

Ross, L. (1996) 'Teaching spiritual care to nurses.' *Nurse Education Today 16*, 38–43.

Scott, E. and Bowen, B. (1997) 'Multidisciplinary collaborative care planning.' *Nursing Standard 12*, 1, 39–42.

Simsen, B. (1985) 'Spiritual needs and resources in illness and hospitalisation.' Unpublished MSc thesis, Manchester: University of Manchester.

South Yorkshire NHS Workforce Development Confederation (2003) 'Caring for the spirit: a strategy for the chaplaincy and spiritual healthcare workforce.' Available from: www.southyorkshire.nhs.uk/chaplaincy/documents/Workforce_Strategy.pdf Accessed 3/3/06.

Stoll, R. (1979) 'Guidelines for spiritual assessment.' *American Journal of Nursing 79*, 1574–1577.

Taylor, E.J. (2002) *Spiritual Care, Nursing Theory, Research and Practice.* New Jersey; Prentice Hall.

Whipp, M. (2001) 'Discerning the spirits: theological audit in health care organizations.' In H. Orchard (ed.) (2001) *Spirituality in Health Care Contexts*, 57–70. London: Jessica Kingsley Publishers.

Further reading

These texts will develop your insight into the issues surrounding the provision of spiritual care. They will clarify how spiritual needs can be addressed within a systematic framework.

Johnson, C.P. (2001) 'Assessment tools: are they an effective approach to implementing spiritual health care within the NHS?' *Accident and Emergency Nursing 9*, 177–186.

McSherry, W. and Ross, L. (2002) 'Dilemmas of spiritual assessment: considerations for nursing practice.' *Journal of Advanced Nursing 38*, 5, 479–488.

Robinson, S., Kendrick, K. and Brown, A. (2003) *Spirituality and the Practice of Healthcare*, 92–122. Houndsmill: Palgrave Macmillan.

Speck, P. (2005) 'The evidence base for spiritual care.' *Nurisng Management 12*, 6, 28–31.

Taylor, E.J. (2002) *Spiritual Care, Nursing Theory, Research and Practice*, 103–157. New Jersey: Prentice Hall.

CHAPTER 5

Barriers Influencing the Provision of Spiritual Care

Introduction

This chapter focuses upon the intrinsic barriers (within the individual) and extrinsic barriers (within the health care situation) that may impede health care professionals' ability to provide spiritual care. The chapter will explore in detail the barriers that exist in practice, presenting some strategies and solutions that may empower health care professionals better to meet an individual's spiritual needs. Case studies are used to generate a deeper awareness and insight into the barriers identified that result in spiritual needs remaining unmet.

Activity 5.1

Using material explored earlier in this book, can you identify any barriers that may prevent health care professionals from addressing or meeting their patients' spiritual needs?

Having reflected upon the case studies presented in earlier chapters, you may have identified several points such as a lack of privacy, fear or ignorance. On closer inspection of your list, you may note that the barriers can be placed into different categories: those that arise from within the health care professional or patient/service user; those concerned with communication; and a further selection that appear on initial reflection to be beyond the control of the health care professional or patient. These barriers will now be explored in greater detail (Box 5.1).

Box 5.1 The two main categories of barriers

Intrinsic

The word 'intrinsic' is used in this context to mean any factor arising within an individual that may affect the provision of spiritual care.

Extrinsic

The word 'extrinsic' is used to describe factors that arise beyond the control of an individual, which prevent or inhibit the provision of spiritual care.

Identifying the barriers

The growing realization that health care professionals can play a fundamental role in the provision of spiritual care has witnessed a proliferation in the amount of published material discussing this issue. This is evident in Box 2.1, Chapter 2.

CAUTION

When reviewing the literature concerning health care professionals' ability to provide spiritual care, the professions are at risk of being dogmatic. Many articles published suggest that health care professionals should be providing spiritual care irrespective of patients' or service users' wishes. This tendency towards being over-prescriptive must be considered when examining the barriers that may prevent health care professionals from providing spiritual care, because such dogmatism may be unjustified.

As the 'caution' indicates, health care could be accused of being over-prescriptive in its approach to spiritual care if it does not exercise sensitivity and flexibility. It is all too easy to legislate for a particular action or manner of conduct without having an appreciation of the full picture. This point is highlighted by a line that appears in the discussion section of an article by Taylor, Highfield and Amenta (1994, p.485): 'However, the somewhat moderate responses to the Likert items indicated these nurses' commitment to, or confidence about, spiritual care is not as strong as could be.' This quotation appears judgemental and extremely prescriptive, critical of nurses' practice in relation to their ability and confidence in meeting patients' spiritual needs. However, Soeken and Carson (1987, p.610) write:

> Meeting the spiritual needs of patients can be uncomfortable for the nurse. Several reasons for such discomforts include embarrassment, the belief that it is not the nurse's role, lack of training, and lack of own spiritual resources.

This quotation seems more balanced, emphasizing that the provision of spiritual care is not simple and straightforward because there are many factors that must be considered. A comparison of Soeken and Carson's quotation with your own list of barriers may reveal similarities.

Research undertaken by a wide range of health care professionals has revealed barriers similar to those identified by Soeken and Carson. Ross (1994, 1997) identified that barriers could be nurse or patient related, profession related, or environmentally related. McSherry (1997) highlighted barriers similar in nature, describing them as economic, educational, environmental or personal in origin. Interestingly, these barriers still exist despite all the attempts to raise the profile of spiritual care and integrate it within care delivery. These barriers are not just specific to nursing. McColl (2000, p.225), writing on the subject of spirituality within occupational therapy practice, recognizes the fears and anxieties that practitioners face: 'After all, if we did Do something or encouraged a client to Do something of a spiritual nature and it backfired, how could we defend ourselves?'

Achieving positive spiritual care

Figure 5.1 illustrates how the successful provision of spiritual care is dependent upon three key areas – the health care professional, the patient/service user, and the economic and environmental context in which spiritual care is provided. It is suggested that for spiritual care to be effective all these three areas must be working in relative harmony. Barriers manifesting themselves in any of these areas will result in the patient's or service user's spiritual needs not necessarily being met. Intrinsic and extrinsic barriers to providing spiritual care will now be discussed in more detail.

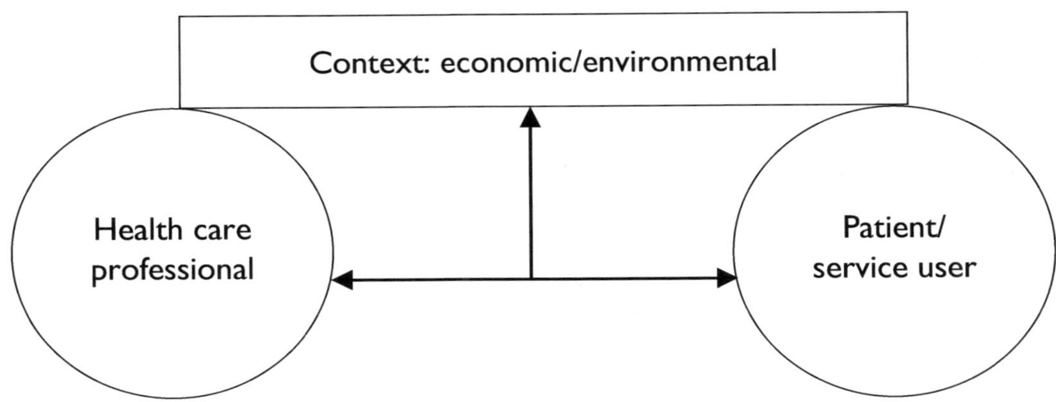

Figure 5.1: The three areas in which barriers may occur

Intrinsic barriers

> I would probably rather tell you about my sex life than about my spiritual life. And I'm fairly sure you would be more scandalized to find a Bible at the bottom of my briefcase than a copy of the *Kama Sutra.* (Allen 1991, p.52)

Charlotte Allen's quotation highlights the deeply personal aspects of spirituality, indicating that there are many personal barriers (intrinsic) that prevent us from addressing this dimension of care with individuals. It would seem that in today's society individuals feel more comfortable talking about sexuality and elimination than about spiritual matters. Implicit in the quotation is the notion that barriers in the provision of spiritual care may not only originate from within the patient, but also from within the nurse or health care professional. The provision of spiritual care is an exchange of energy – an encounter – between two individuals: the health care professional and the service user, the doctor and the patient, or the patient and his or her own spiritual leader. Therefore, barriers in the exchange of this energy may arise from within any of these key individuals.

The intrinsic barriers that may prevent the provision of spiritual care are not specific to the patient. Figure 5.1 shows that the provision of spiritual care is a two-way process between the patient/service user and the health care professional (Clark *et al.* 1991). Therefore, an intrinsic barrier may develop within either the health care professional or the patient/service user, preventing spiritual needs from being addressed. Some of the intrinsic barriers that may arise are listed in Box 5.2. Researchers, as outlined earlier, have identified several of these barriers (McSherry 1997; Waugh 1992).

Intrinsic barriers may be associated with our own personal belief systems, which may be in conflict with that of the patient. For example, our attitudes towards certain religious groups may be prejudiced by the beliefs and values we have acquired through socialization. Another example may be the attitudes we have towards different sections in society, such as the social stigma attached to HIV and AIDS or the misconceptions associated with asylum seekers, and the rise in 'Islamaphobia'. Other barriers may occur because of our inability to communicate effectively with patients or our service users. The barriers listed in Box 5.2 are now discussed in detail.

Box 5.2 Intrinsic barriers

Inability to communicate through illness or loss of senses

Ambiguity

Lack of knowledge in the area of spirituality

Patient not aware of the concept of spiritual need

Sensitive area – too personal for nurses to address

Own personal beliefs and values

Emotionally demanding and fear-provoking

Fears – mismanagement

Prejudices

Inability to communicate through illness or loss of senses

McCavery (1985, p.130) stresses the importance of good communication in providing spiritual care: 'In many ways, spiritual care is subjective, and its success rests upon the meaning of conversations between individual patients and nurse.'

Working from this quotation, a major obstacle in the provision of spiritual care is a breakdown in the channels of communication. Ross (1994) presents several conditions that can impede communication such as aphasia (loss of speech), or any other problem associated with the loss of a sense such as sight or hearing (see Case study 5.2). The inability to communicate effectively can result in an individual being unable to express a spiritual need, and the nurse being unable to assess or interpret the situation. The overall results of such situations may see the patient's or service user's spiritual needs remaining unrecognized and consequently unmet. This inability to communicate effectively can mean that the patient and nurse become frustrated. Such situations are not easy to resolve, as there are no easy solutions. The health care professional may use a variety of techniques to try to establish what the individual needs, such as writing needs down, using word charts, or even enlisting an interpreter to translate a patient's or service user's needs.

Another aspect of communication that can prove problematic is communicating effectively with individuals who may not have the intellectual development or capacity to think abstractly, such as young children, individuals with severe learning disabilities or clients with organic brain disease such as dementia (Case study 5.1).

This case study stresses the importance of providing spiritual care that is appropriate and at the correct level for individuals to comprehend. Sommer (1989, p.231) highlights some of the difficulties practitioners may face when attending to the spiritual needs of dying children:

> Children can readily sense when adults are uncomfortable with a topic of discussion or a situation. Whereas healthy children like to express their uniqueness, sick and dying children like to find ways of blending in with the crowd.

The issues identified in this quotation are certainly evident in Samantha's situation (Case study 5.1). The importance of good communication and interpersonal skills in managing such situations is paramount. If barriers exist that prevent channels of communication, then our human condition may result in avoidance of the situation. Samantha's situation is difficult, with the potential for it to be emotionally demanding and exhausting. Such situations challenge and drain the emotional and spiritual reserves of the most experienced practitioners.

Ambiguity

Ambiguity is when uncertainty or a lack of insight into situations prevents either the nurse or the patient from entering into a therapeutic relationship. Numerous reasons for this may exist and it is not unique to the spiritual

Case study 5.1 How to proceed

Samantha is eight years of age and diagnosed with an inoperable terminal brain tumour. Samantha has been told about her condition and seems to avoid any mention of the issue. She keeps repeating time and again, 'I do not want to die, Mammy'.

What do you feel are the intrinsic issues that may be barriers in providing adequate spiritual care?

dimension. However, because of the deeply personal nature of spirituality, ambiguity may arise when the health care professional and patient/service user have contrasting belief systems and personalities. This can be illustrated by the situation where a health care professional – for example, a nurse who does not have any belief in God – is asked to be primary nurse for a patient who is a practising Christian attending a very Evangelical church. At every opportunity the patient tries to convert the nurse. This situation may arouse a great deal of insecurity, frustration and vulnerability within the nurse. The result may be that the nurse feels that his or her personal belief system is being challenged and, where possible, the nurse may avoid making any meaningful contact with the patient. Similarly, a nurse may have strong beliefs about the sanctity of life, and may decline to participate in the surgical procedure of termination of pregnancy.

The need for health care professionals to provide care that does not project their own personal beliefs onto patients or service users is evident. Within my own profession of nursing, two cases of Registered Nurses being brought before the Nursing and Midwifery Conduct Committee (formally the United Kingdom Central Council for Nursing and Midwifery) for professional misconduct have been documented (Castledine 2005, p.745; Cobb 2001, p.74). These cases serve as a stark warning for all health care professionals about the need for self-awareness.

Lack of knowledge in the area of spirituality

Ambiguity may also arise when the service user or health care professional does not know what is meant by the term 'spiritual need'. On a cautionary note, just because an individual is not familiar with the language of spirituality does not mean that spiritual needs will go unmet. Draper and McSherry (2002, p.1) write:

> We suggest that adequate conceptual vocabulary already exists to enable us to understand and support them (or at least to try) – this is the vocabulary of loss, grief, fear, anxiety, hope, despair, joy and realization, we can see no advantage in superimposing a further vocabulary of spirituality.

There is an urgent need for health care professionals to research more fully patients' and health care professionals' understanding of these terms. However, as Swinton and Narayanasamy (2002, p.158) correctly point out:

> ...we propose that it is reasonable to suggest that the spiritual dimension not only exists, but also should be taken seriously by all nurses who profess to offer holistic care. To dismiss the universality of spirituality summarily on the grounds of one study would appear to be unreasonable.

This quotation rightly alerts all health care professionals to the fact that there may well be numerous ways of defining spirituality, and that just because the language of spirituality may not always be recognized at a personal level by patients or service users does not mean the concept is obsolete. For ambiguity to be removed, health care professionals need to be introspective, being aware of their own personal beliefs, values and, importantly, prejudices. Reflecting upon practice or critical incidents that are encountered in relation to spiritual matters will enable practitioners to evaluate their own emotions and feelings, formulating strategies that will allow them perhaps to cope better or adjust their practice should similar situations be encountered in the future (McColl 2000; McSherry 1996, 2004).

Sensitive area – too personal for health care professionals to address

McSherry (1997) asked nurses to provide some qualitative responses into what they perceived were the main barriers in the provision of spiritual care. Several of the nurses surveyed indicated that the area of spirituality was too sensitive to be addressed by nurses. In fact, McSherry's (2004) qualitative study, which included a broad range of health care professionals, confirmed this earlier finding. The notion of sensitivity included the nurses' or health care professionals' own fears of mismanagement of delicate and often deeply personal situations. Harrison (1993) highlighted a particular concern related to over-involvement in situations one cannot handle – 'getting out of one's depth'. Another aspect of sensitivity is the fear of knowing what to say when a patient or service user asks an awkward existential question, such as 'Why me?' or 'What have I done to deserve this?' This type of searching can challenge the health care professional, bringing into question his or her own personal spirituality or philosophies surrounding life, death and religion. It would appear that spiritual care extends health care beyond task focus and demands health care professionals to give of themselves and develop relationships, not just to perform tasks.

Emotionally demanding and fear-provoking

The information presented in relation to the intrinsic barriers indicates that there is an emotional cost or labour involved in the provision of spiritual care in that it can be emotionally and spiritually demanding. Tony Walter (2002, p.138), in his article titled 'Spirituality in palliative care: opportunity or burden?', raises some fundamental points about the assumption that all nurses or health care professionals can meet patients' spiritual needs. He concludes his work with the following recommendation that has poignancy for all advocating spiritual care:

> With careful attention being paid to each individual patient, and with knowledge of what each member of the team can and cannot offer, it may be possible to find someone who can accompany each patient at least a little of the way. But it need not be me. This should relieve each member of the team of the burden of feeling obliged to accompany each and every patient.

The material presented throughout this book indicates that many aspects associated with spirituality are deeply personal; indeed, some issues are emotionally charged, such as those pertaining to religion or matters concerning the sanctity of life. These areas can be extremely difficult for health care professionals to address because they can arouse the personal fears that shape our attitudes and opinions. The fear of mismanagement or making a wrong judgement in difficult situations can lead to avoidance or denial that a patient or service user has a particular spiritual need(s) that requires attention. Case study 5.2 shows how the health care professional may have to play an arbitrary role – acting as advocate for the spiritual needs of the patient as well as being sensitive to the spiritual needs of immediate family and friends. Salladay and McDonnell (1989, p.543) write:

> A skilled patient advocate is a nurse who is first able and willing to set aside personal agendas and unit politics to participate with patients in their search for meaning during times that patients may be suffering, vulnerable, or frustrated.

This quotation implies that the role of advocate is fundamental when supporting patients or service users in their decision making. Read Case study 5.2, paying particular attention to those factors that may place an emotional burden upon the nurse or health care professional.

Case study 5.2 In whose interest?

Mr Francis was admitted to the ward having suffered a very dense left-sided CVA (cerebrovascular accident, or stroke). For two days he was deeply unconscious and unresponsive, and was given intravenous fluids for hydration. Several days passed and slowly Mr Francis gained consciousness and became more alert. Prior to admission, he had been a very active man who had had an excellent quality of life, free of any major illness or hospitalization. Mr Francis' wife and family stayed with him and supported him throughout the acute phase of the illness. Mr Francis' condition improved, and the process of rehabilitation was initiated. It soon became apparent that Mr Francis was aphasic, having a marked dysphagia. It was decided by the medical and nursing staff, in consultation with Mr Francis and his family, to pass a fine bore nasogastric tube and to commence enteral feeding. However, Mr Francis showed dissatisfaction with this by pulling out the tube. Again the tube was passed, and again Mr Francis pulled out the tube, to the displeasure of his family.

The nurses and consultant caring for Mr Francis discussed the matter with him, and it emerged that he did not want to be fed. However, when his family were present, he would change his mind in an attempt to keep the peace. Mr Francis' family were rightly concerned that he would possibly starve to death, and asked for a gastrostomy tube to be inserted. Mr Francis agreed and consented to have the procedure performed. Several days later, he pulled out the gastrostomy tube and categorically refused to have it reinserted. Again when approached by the consultant and nursing staff, Mr Francis indicated non-verbally that he did not want the gastrostomy tube reinserting. The consultant explained the situation in detail, informing him of the consequences of his decision, and that he would die if he were left without nutritional support. Mr Francis was adamant in his decision, and even persuasion from his family failed. Consequently, Mr Francis died some days later.

Having read the case study, you have probably identified correctly that there are many ethical issues operating in this situation. With respect to Mr Francis' spiritual needs, he has come to a conscious decision that life is no longer worth living. There is a need to be aware that depression is a major complication affecting individuals who have suffered a stroke. Depression had been assessed for and excluded in Mr Francis' situation. However, he is faced with a dilemma – 'torn between the devil and the deep blue sea'. He is possibly thinking that his quality of life will never be the same. Yet Mr Francis is conscious of the needs of his family and the impact that his decision will have upon them. The case study indicates that Mr Francis' family are faced with the potential death of a loved one. It would appear that Mr Francis has made a conscious decision to die by not wanting to be enterally fed. However, he seeks to keep the peace and placate his family by following their wishes and instructions when they are present. In such situations, the nurse may experience divided loyalties – wanting to act as advocate for the patient but at the same time appreciating the helplessness, grief and spiritual distress that loved ones may be feeling when faced with such dilemmas.

These situations can place an emotional and spiritual strain upon all those involved. The health care professional may need to act as an arbitrator/advocate between the patient and their family. Disagreement may occur between health care workers as to the appropriateness of the course of action chosen. The final outcome should be determined and made by the patient or service user themselves (where possible) since it is their spiritual needs that are paramount, overriding the needs of others involved in the situation.

The antagonism and division one can experience in such situations can deplete one's own emotional and spiritual reserve – causing anxiety and fear. The ever-growing threat of complaint and litigation can further compound such situations. Questions like 'Did we take the appropriate course of action?' or 'Did we act in the best interests of individuals?' may be asked, especially when situations are complex, involving and affecting the perceptions and opinions of several individuals.

Extrinsic factors

This section will focus upon the category of barriers termed extrinsic – you may recall that these barriers are those external to an individual. Read Activity 5.2 and answer the question that follows.

Activity 5.2

Mr Singh Bhuller is a practising Sikh. The wearing of religious symbols and prayer are fundamental. Mr Singh is concerned that his customs and daily rituals will not be maintained while in hospital. You are the admitting nurse working on a busy, general surgical ward. Can you identify any extrinsic barriers that may prevent Mr Singh from observing his religious practices while in your care?

You may have identified several extrinsic or environmental barriers that may prevent Mr Singh from maintaining his religious customs and practices, while making sense of his illness and hospitalization:

- lack of personal space
- environmental distractions/interruptions
- prayer heard by other patients/staff on the ward
- staff too busy to facilitate
- perhaps religious needs not adequately assessed upon admission
- uncertainty concerning religious needs of Mr Singh.

Some of these barriers are associated with lack of privacy. Others are determined by management or organizational structures such as insufficient staff, the way that patient care is organized, the resources available to address Mr Singh's spiritual needs, or lack of time due to the busy nature of the ward. All these barriers will determine the amount of time the nurses will be able to devote to Mr Singh's general and spiritual care. Box 5.3 presents a list of extrinsic barriers that have been identified by researchers (McSherry 1998; Ross 1994). Compare this against your own list, noting any similarities or differences.

As indicated earlier, there is now more emphasis placed on all health care establishments providing care to diverse and wide-ranging client groups to address and support the spiritual needs of all individuals – both consumers and providers. This reversal in trends has seen spirituality placed firmly on management's operational agendas. This is evident in a letter written by Edward Lewis, Chief Officer of the Hospitals Chaplaincies Council and sent to Chief Executives of National Health Service Trusts and to chaplaincy networks, concerning chaplains/spiritual care givers and the Data Protection Act:

> If Trusts fail to set up an adequate system for allowing patients to be asked about their spiritual care whilst in hospital and to register their consent for this information to be passed on, they could themselves be liable under The Human Rights Act 1998, should a patient claim that s/he was denied the right enshrined in Article 9 of the ECHR to manifest his or her religion, in worship, teaching, practice and observance. (DH 2003, p.32)

This quotation sends a very clear message to all managers – indeed all involved in the provision of health care – highlighting the fundamental right of all individuals to express and be supported in fulfilling their religious and spiritual needs. It also suggests that Trusts should be sensible in the way that they work with chaplaincy departments in managing issues of access to patients and service users and dealing with the problematic area of gaining consent.

Box 5.3 Extrinsic barriers

Organizational and management

Environmental distractions resulting in loss of privacy

Economic constraints

Shortages of staff

Lack of time

Educational issues

Reduced length of stay in hospital

Not directly relevant to area of practice

Prevailing opinions within society

Organizational and management

If health care professionals are to provide effective spiritual care, then there is a need for management to address many of the extrinsic barriers identified. The growing evidence addressing the spiritual dimension needs to be reviewed and a model of best practice devised, implemented and evaluated at local and national levels. Management needs to accept some responsibility for the provision of spiritual care. This responsibility and accountability has been made explicit in recent policy guidelines and directives (DH 2001, 2003; SEHD 2002). The importance of providing an environment and climate in which a patient's or service user's spiritual or religious beliefs can be addressed should now be the norm rather than an optional extra. Therefore, health care professionals should alert management to any environmental, economic or educational barriers that prevent them from implementing or addressing patients', service users' or staffs' spiritual needs satisfactorily, thus influencing the overall standard of care provided and the environment in which staff have to provide care. However, caution needs to be exercised because managerial and organizational constraints could be used as an excuse for not getting involved.

Environmental distractions resulting in loss of privacy

Environmental barriers are ultimately determined by the context in which all care is to be provided. In the past, acute sector care was provided on large 'Nightingale wards' where it was hard to maintain privacy or personal space. Privacy in such situations is gained by pulling round a curtain screen. This screen does preserve dignity but does not prevent personal conversations from being overheard. In such situations, patients may not divulge personal information for fear that neighbouring patients are listening. It is hard to maintain confidentiality under such circumstances. Such problems may be overcome if the number of quiet rooms where patients could be counselled privately were increased.

It could be argued that many modern hospitals and health care settings are now much better suited to the needs of patients and service users in respect of preserving dignity and affording privacy. Many areas now within the primary, secondary and tertiary sectors have facilities in which patients and service users can be counselled in private, keeping distractions and interruptions to a minimum. Furthermore, there now seems to be greater emphases on keeping patients and service users within their own homes, with outreach teams supporting patients/service users to live as independently as possible.

This shift in emphasis from acute to primary care may enhance the provision of spiritual care by reducing some of the environmental deficits providing it is suitably resourced.

Economic constraints

Possibly the greatest obstacle in the provision of spiritual care, within the acute sectors, is lack of time and the restricted availability of staff (McSherry 1997). The contemporary health care system has changed drastically, witnessing an increased in-patient and service user expectation alongside a dramatic reduction in numbers of many of the health care professions due to inability to either recruit or retain. The result has seen health care staff providing care in situations that are highly stressful and demanding. In such situations, spiritual care is seen as a low priority when contrasted against other more life-saving situations. The qualified nurse or health care professional cannot be expected to provide spiritual care if he or she does not have the time to communicate or listen effectively.

Shortages of staff

It could be argued that the government has responded to this urgent need with recent pay incentives and the publication of documents like *Making a Difference: Strengthening the nursing, Midwifery and Health Visiting Contribution to Health and Health Care* (DH 1999). More recently, we have seen the introduction of *The NHS Knowledge and Skills Framework (NHS KSF) and Development Review Process* (DH 2005). However, it is my firm belief that these are not long-term solutions but rather short-term remedies to try to reverse the worrying trend that afflicts the delivery of health and social care in many situations. The accumulative effect of recent trends – for example, shortage of nurses, junior doctors and many other health care professionals means that there is now over-reliance upon agency or locum staff – brings into question the overall quality of care provided. Therefore, when health care professionals report that they are too busy to provide spiritual care, this probably reflects the reality of the situation in which they work.

Lack of time

Cynics may offer a counter-argument by stating that spiritual care is not something different from the 'general care' provided by health care professionals. Therefore, the claims that 'we are too busy' or 'do not have sufficient time or staff' are redundant. Management are aware that to deliver a high standard of care requires commitment from staff who are highly trained and skilled within their chosen specialty. The same principle must be applied to the provision of spiritual care. The spiritual needs of patients and service users will not be adequately addressed if they are left to chance.

CAUTION

The lack of time could be seen as an excuse for not becoming involved. Spiritual care can be provided within the context of general care. The interactions that take place when bathing a patient or dressing a wound can be used to build trust and offer spiritual support.

Educational issues

Educational debates surrounding the spiritual dimension are addressed in more detail in Chapter 7. However, one major barrier that has been identified by numerous research studies is that health care professionals feel or are inadequately prepared to meet the spiritual needs of their patients or service users (Boutell and Bozett 1990; Narayanasamy 1993; Waugh 1992). McSherry's (1997) survey revealed that some nurses did not feel confident in addressing a patient's spiritual needs because of a lack of insight or knowledge of this aspect of care. Almost a decade on and health care professionals were still indicating that they were not adequately prepared to deal with spiritual issues (McSherry 2004).

Reduced length of stay in hospital

Within the acute sector, the average stay in hospital is around 48 hours. This has been greatly reduced by advances in surgical procedures, screening and new investigative techniques. These advances have to be viewed positively since they reduce the stress placed on individuals as a result of extensive hospitalization. However, this reduction in the length of stay may mean patients' and service users' spiritual needs are left unmet. Rapid turnover or throughput of patients means the opportunity may not exist for health care professionals to establish a trusting relationship in which a patient or service user may reveal a spiritual need. Likewise, health care professionals may be too concerned or preoccupied with outcome measures and bed occupancy figures, resulting in spiritual care being afforded low priority. Turner (1996, p.60) recognizes that this dilemma may also be affecting hospice care:

> Even in hospice care the process of bureaucratisation has produced a growing preoccupation with throughput, outcomes and cost-effectiveness, hence a concern for doing with little or no emphasis on being.

These concerns may not always affect care that is provided within the community or primary care settings, where practitioners have the opportunity and time to establish relationships that may extend over a period of weeks, and, in the case of some chronic illnesses, months or years. Likewise, nurses working with individuals with learning disabilities may have the opportunity to establish a meaningful relationship with their clients or users of a service over an extended period of time. The opportunity to develop such relationships can prove very rewarding for the client and the health care professional since both can learn and grow spiritually together (Balkizas and O'Hare 1994; Males and Boswell 1990).

Not directly relevant to area of practice

The relevance of nursing staff – indeed any health care professional intervening and addressing patients' spiritual needs – has been identified as a potential barrier (McCavery 1985; McSherry 1997). For example, health care professionals working within certain specialties such as intensive care units may find it difficult to provide spiritual care to individuals who are unconscious and being ventilated. Likewise, health care professionals working within rehabilitation units may find it difficult to provide spiritual care to individuals in a persistent vegetative state. The barriers originate from the inability to communicate effectively in that communication may be one-sided and perceived as ineffective. Read Case study 5.3 and reflect upon how you might feel if you were the nurse caring for John.

It is easy to assume that individuals who are unconscious or unresponsive do not require spiritual care. This assumption usually stems from our inability to interact with the patient in a meaningful manner. Even the most experienced of health care professionals may find it difficult to communicate with ease in such circumstances. However, these circumstances should not prevent one from providing patient-centred and holistic care, accepting that behind the seemingly motionless exterior lies a human being in whom resides a spirit that requires nurturing and caring.

Case study 5.3

John, a 21-year-old mechanic, was knocked off his motor bike and sustained severe head injuries. Surgery was performed to remove a large subdural haematoma. John never regained consciousness and was diagnosed as being in a persistent vegetative state. After several months in the neurosurgical ward, John was transferred to a rehabilitation unit for intensive stimulation and rehabilitation. Prior to his accident, John used to enjoy socializing with his colleagues and friends. He was a keen musician, playing guitar in a local rock band.

Some health care professionals may question the relevance and appropriateness of tinkering in this aspect of individuals' lives, suggesting that spiritual issues should be addressed and dealt with by the hospital chaplain or the individual's own spiritual/religious leader. However, this is a grave misconception since it assumes that spirituality is solely concerned with the religious. This approach towards spirituality could be seen as a defence mechanism that prevents health care professionals from being involved in an aspect of care that can be challenging and threatening. The literature indicates that nurses in particular are in a prime position to attend to the spiritual needs of their patients because of their 24-hour responsibilities. Merely to state that the spiritual dimension is not our responsibility can be construed as 'passing the buck'.

Prevailing opinions within society

Allen (1991, p.52) implies that forces operating within society, or indeed within the nursing profession, may be a major obstacle in the provision of spiritual care. Individual health care professionals may not want to be seen as nonconforming – going against popular opinion and belief. Involvement in an individual's spiritual care may result in other health care professionals making value judgements about a colleague's motives. Some may see a health care professional who attends to the spiritual needs of patients as a fanatic – a 'Bible basher' – when in reality all they are trying to do is provide total patient care. In such instances, the health care professional may provide spiritual care in secrecy or, sadly, the health care professional may stop attending to the spiritual needs of patients or service users because of fear of reprisal or recrimination. These anxieties are highlighted by Aveyard (1995, p.44) when discussing the concept of self-disclosure within teaching: 'But on the rare occasions when I have referred to instances relating to my faith, I sense that some students feel that it is inappropriate.'

Therefore, social desirability may be a force that inhibits the provision of spiritual care. Yet, ideally, we should see all practitioners, regardless of race, creed, colour or religion, attending to the spiritual needs of patients and service users. In an ideal world, this would mean we do not make value judgements about other individuals but instead use tolerance and common sense. There needs to be a sense of proportion. Likewise, we would not want individuals with strong religious beliefs trying to convert, or preaching to vulnerable patients or service users.

Activity 5.3

Read this chapter again thinking specifically about any strategies or measures you could use to try to address some of these barriers within yourself or your practice environment.

No easy solutions

As indicated, it is all too easy to become prescriptive, stating that health care professionals should be providing spiritual care without giving due thought and attention to the demands and pressures that many encounter in the course of their practice. However, it is also easy to declare that we cannot do anything to remove these political and economic barriers until the wastage, attrition and recruitment problems that shroud health care are resolved. If we adopt this approach, then many patients' and service users' spiritual needs in our care will be left unmet. Box 5.4 presents some steps that we may take to overcome the barriers that prevent health care professionals from providing spiritual care.

There is a need for us to inform management of shortfalls in staff levels that impinge on all aspects of care. We need to develop insight into our own spirituality and spiritual needs. By becoming spiritually aware, we will be in a stronger position to recognize similar needs within our patients, service users and colleagues. We need to be aware of our own personal fears and prejudices that may influence our attitudes to this dimension of care. By exploring our own personal beliefs and values, we may better be able to tolerate and accept that we are all unique with diverse belief and value systems. Schoenbeck (1994) suggests that the key to effective spiritual care is respectfulness of the patient's or individual's belief system.

Box 5.4 Steps we can take to remove the barriers

Intrinsic

Self-awareness. Become more introspective, reflecting upon our own beliefs and attitudes, values. Think about our own spirituality. Question our attitudes to different groups, situations.

Tolerance and patience. Respect those with different cultural, ethnic or religious principles instead of making value judgements.

Extrinsic

Inform. Make management aware of any obstacles that inhibit us from delivering the quality of care that we strive to provide. This may be the lack of a quiet room on the ward or unit in which to talk privately with patients/service users, or drawing attention to poor staffing levels and skills mix.

Resources. Be aware of who the chaplains are and the service that they provide. We need to be aware of the resources at our disposal that can assist us in providing spiritual care, such as information leaflets or books that offer insight into the customs and practices of different religions. Know where to contact an interpreter if required.

Conclusion

This chapter has introduced you to the numerous barriers, intrinsic and extrinsic, that may prevent health care professionals from delivering spiritual care. It has been stressed that there are many variables that must be considered before we accuse health care of failing to provide spiritual care. If health care professions adopt a judgemental and prescriptive attitude towards the delivery of spiritual care, then they could be accused of double standards. This would be so because they would be failing to acknowledge the many pressures, political and economic, that may prevent practitioners from attending to their patients' or service users' spiritual needs. However, it is suggested that there are many measures we can adopt in order to remove some of the barriers that prevent us from providing spiritual care. By far the greatest measure we can take is to develop our own spiritual awareness, which will enable us to remove many of the intrinsic barriers. Once we have put our own house in order, then we can turn our attention to the extrinsic barriers that exist within practice.

References

Allen, C. (1991) 'The inner light.' *Nursing Standard 5*, 20, 52–53.

Aveyard, B. (1995) 'A question of faith.' *Nursing Standard 9*, 5, 44.

Balkizas, D. and O'Hare, M. (1994) 'The healing hand of God.' *Nursing Standard 9*, 9, 46–47.

Boutell, K.A. and Bozett, F.W. (1990) 'Nurses' assessment of patients' spirituality: continuing education implications.' *Journal of Continuing Education in Nursing 21*, 4, 172–176.

Castledine, G. (2005) 'Senior nurse who demeaned the spiritual beliefs of patients and staff.' *British Journal of Nursing 14*, 14, 745.

Clark, C.C., Cross, J.R., Deane, D.M. and Lowry, L.W. (1991) 'Spirituality: integral to quality care.' *Holistic Nursing Practice 5*, 3, 67–76.

Cobb, M. (2001) 'Walking on water? The moral foundation of chaplaincy.' In H. Orchard (ed.) (2001) *Spirituality in Health Care Contexts*, 73–83. London: Jessica Kingsley Publishers.

Department of Health (DH) (1999) *Making a Difference: Strengthening the Nursing, Midwifery and Health Visiting Contribution to Health and Health Care.* London: HMSO.

Department of Health (2001) *Your Guide to the NHS.* London: Department of Health.

Department of Health (2003) *NHS Chaplaincy: Meeting the Religious and Spiritual Needs of Patients and Staff.* London: Department of Health.

Department of Health (2005) *The NHS Knowledge and Skills Framework (NHS KSF) and Development Review Process.* Available from: www.dh.gov.uk/assetRoot/04/10/86/44/04108644.pdf Accessed 1/11/05.

Draper, P. and McSherry, W. (2002) 'A critical review of spirituality and spiritual assessment.' *Journal of Advanced Nursing 39*, 1, 1–2.

Harrison, J. (1993) 'Spirituality and nursing practice.' *Journal of Clinical Nursing 2*, 211–217.

Males, J. and Boswell, C. (1990) 'Spiritual needs of people with a mental handicap.' *Nursing Standard 4*, 48, 35–37.

McCavery, R. (1985) 'Spiritual care in acute illness.' In O. McGilloway and F. Myco (eds) *Nursing and Spiritual Care.* London: Harper and Row.

McColl, M.A. (2000) 'Spirit, occupation and disability.' *The Canadian Journal of Occupational Therapy 67*, 4, 217–228.

McSherry, W. (1996) 'Raising the spirits.' *Nursing Times 92*, 3, 48–49.

McSherry, W. (1997) 'A descriptive survey of nurses' perceptions of spirituality and spiritual care.' Unpublished MPhil thesis, Hull: University of Hull.

McSherry, W. (1998) 'Nurses' perceptions of spirituality and spiritual care.' *Nursing Standard 13*, 4, 36–40.

McSherry, W. (2004) 'The meaning of spirituality and spiritual care: an investigation of health care professionals', patients' and public's perceptions.' Unpublished PhD thesis, Leeds: Leeds Metropolitan University.

Narayanasamy, A. (1993) 'Nurses' awareness and educational preparation in meeting their patients' spiritual needs.' *Nurse Education Today 13*, 3, 196–201.

Ross, L. (1994) 'Spiritual care: the nurse's role.' *Nursing Standard 8*, 33, 33–37.

Ross, L. (1997) 'The nurse's role in assessing and responding to patients' spiritual needs.' *International Journal of Palliative Nursing 3*, 1, 37–42.

Salladay, S.A. and McDonnell, M.M. (1989) 'Spiritual care, ethical choices and patient advocacy.' *Nursing Clinics of North America 24*, 2, 543–549.

Schoenbeck, S.L. (1994) 'Called to care: addressing the spiritual needs of patients.' *Journal of Practical Nursing 44*, 3, 19–23.

Scottish Executive Health Department (SEHD) (2002) *Guidelines on Chaplaincy and Spiritual Care in the NHS in Scotland* (NHS HDL (2002) 76). Edinburgh; Scottish Executive.

Soeken, K.L. and Carson, V.B. (1987) 'Responding to the spiritual needs of the chronically ill.' *Nursing Clinics of North America 22*, 3, 603–611.

Sommer, D.R. (1989) 'The spiritual needs of dying children.' *Issues in Comprehensive Paediatric Nursing 12*, 2/3, 225–233.

Swinton, J. and Narayanasamy, A. (2002) 'Response to: A critical view of spirituality and spiritual assessment by P. Draper and W. McSherry.' *Journal of Advanced Nursing 39*, 1–2, *Journal of Advanced Nursing 40*, 2, 158–160.

Taylor, J.E., Highfield, M. and Amenta, M. (1994) 'Attitudes and beliefs regarding spiritual care.' *Cancer Nursing 17*, 6, 479–487.

Turner, P. (1996) 'Caring more, doing less.' *Nursing Times 92*, 34, 59–60.

Walter, T. (2002) 'Spirituality in palliative care: opportunity or burden?' *Palliative Medicine 16*, 133–139.

Waugh, L.A. (1992) 'Spiritual aspects of nursing: a descriptive study of nurses' perceptions.' Unpublished PhD thesis, Edinburgh: Queen Margaret College.

Further reading

These texts will further develop your understanding of the barriers, intrinsic and extrinsic, that may affect health care professionals' ability to provide spiritual care. These texts are informative and interesting to read. By reflecting upon their content you will gain a deeper insight into many of the issues addressed in the chapter.

Hollins, S. (2005) 'Spirituality and religion: exploring the relationship.' *Nursing Management 12*, 6, 22–26.

Johnson, A. (1998) 'The notion of spiritual care in professional practice.' In M. Cobb and V. Robshaw (1998) *The Spiritual Challenge of Health Care*, 151–166. Edinburgh: Churchill Livingstone.

Kellehear, A. (2002) 'Spiritual care in palliative care: whose job is it?' In B. Rumbold (2002) *Spirituality and Palliative Care: Social and Pastoral Perspectives*, 166–177. Melbourne, Australia: Oxford University Press.

Speck, P. (2005) 'The evidence base for spiritual care.' *Nursing Management 12*, 6, 28–31.

Walter, T. (2002) 'Spirituality in palliative care: opportunity or burden?' *Palliative Medicine 16*, 133–139.

CHAPTER 6

Skills Required to Provide Spiritual Care

Introduction

This chapter will review the different skills health care professionals require in order to assess, plan, implement and evaluate spiritual care. At this stage in the book, you are probably recognizing that the concept of spirituality is subjective, diverse and unique to each individual. The subjective nature of the spiritual dimension means that health care professionals require a broad range of skills for them to overcome many of the barriers that can prevent the provision of spiritual care. By utilizing these skills and developing their own self-awareness, health care professionals will be in a stronger position to act as advocates for their patients, clients or service users who present with spiritual need(s). The chapter demonstrates the need for multidisciplinary and inter-disciplinary collaboration in the provision of spiritual care. It is argued that no single professional group has a monopoly with respect to the spiritual dimension.

In Box 6.1, the quotation from Burnard highlights the subtle nature of spiritual care. It reveals that spiritual care is not easy, and at times is uncomfortable, indeed a challenge. The quotation implies that there are right and wrong methods to be utilized in this aspect of care. Fundamentally, the quotation indicates that the area of spiritual care is a two-way process that can enrich the lives of both the patient and the nurse or health care professional – a term I have called professional enrichment (McSherry 2004). However, if spiritual care is to be effective and the dispirited person and the health care professional are to benefit from the interactions and encounter, then there are certain skills or guiding principles to be followed.

Box 6.1 Food for thought

This, then is the challenge in nursing (health care) the spiritually distressed person: to listen, to accept, to explore and finally, to offer no ready answers. This is clearly a difficult task but a rewarding one. In the end, persons who discover their own meaning and their own reason for believing in what they do will usually be the more satisfied. The nurse's task is not to get in the way of that process taking place. But equally and almost paradoxically, it is the nurse's task to become involved with the dispirited person. The balance between standing back and becoming immersed is a difficult one to achieve. It is also, a very human and important one. (Burnard 1987, p.381)

Identifying the skills

In order to proceed with this chapter, there is a need to identify the skills that may be required by health care professionals to support and facilitate spiritual care. Read the following Case study 6.1 and spend several minutes reflecting upon the skills you would require in order to meet the patient's spiritual needs.

You may have identified several skills that are necessary to support Vincent and meet his spiritual needs. You will have recognized the need for good interpersonal skills in helping you to address Vincent's immediate concerns. The questions that Vincent expresses are existential, questioning his reason for living, indicating that you may require some insight into what constitutes spirituality. A comprehensive list of skills required to enable Vincent to achieve total well-being is given in Box 6.2. It must be stressed that these skills are not used in isolation. The biggest danger of identifying lists is that we assume each skill is separate from the next, not connected or used in conjunction with the others. If you observe skilled practitioners, you will see that they draw upon their knowledge and use all their skills in an integrated manner. The skills and knowledge become an integral part of the person. These skills are drawn upon to resolve an issue or concern. The same principle applies

Case study 6.1 Questioning meaning and purpose

Vincent is 38 years of age and works as a business executive with an international company. He has been married for 10 years and has three young children, all under six. He is a little overweight and smokes around 10 cigarettes per day. His wife has been encouraging him to slow down but with little success. Life operates around Vincent's need to meet deadlines and production targets. Early one morning, he is woken by a tightness around his chest and a pain radiating down his left arm and up into his jaw. His wife phones for an ambulance and Vincent is rushed into hospital diagnosed as a myocardial infarction. You are the nurse responsible for Vincent's care. The day after admission, in conversation he says to you, 'My life will never be the same' and 'What will I do about work and who will support my family?'

when supporting individuals with spiritual needs. The provision of spiritual care must become a natural part of the practitioner's experience or else the care will be fragmented and unnatural – rather like using a checklist when a vehicle has been booked in for an MOT test. McCavery (1985, p.139) alerts us to this fact: 'However, spiritual activity can never be restricted to mere religious practice, nor can spiritual needs be fulfilled successfully in a scientific, planned way.'

Perhaps while examining the skills listed, you may feel that many health care professionals already possess such skills, which are developed to a high standard and used frequently in their clinical practice.

To assume that no health care professionals are able to deal with patients' or service users' spiritual needs is presumptuous and judgemental, bearing in mind the concerns raised by Walter (2002) that not all practitioners may want to be involved or could be involved in the delivery of spiritual care. One cannot generalize and say that health care professionals are not able to meet their patients' or service users' spiritual needs. Such a generalization would be misleading, contradicting current research findings (Harrison 1993; McSherry 1997; Narayanasamy 1993; Waugh 1992). An excerpt from McSherry's thesis (1997, p.127) supports this point, indicating that nurses are recognizing patients presenting with a spiritual need(s):

> Of the nurses surveyed 465 (84.7%) stated that they had encountered a patient(s) with a spiritual need(s). A limitation of this question is that there is no means of identifying how frequently, or how recently the nurse had identified such a need(s). Of the qualified nurses surveyed 219 (39.9%) felt that they were able to meet their patient's spiritual needs. A limitation in relation to this question is that specific needs were not asked for or identified.

However, there is no room for complacency because only a small percentage of qualified nurses felt they were able to meet their patients' spiritual need(s) successfully. In several research studies (McSherry 1997, 2004; Narayanasamy 1993; Waugh 1992), nurses and other health care professionals have asked for more education regarding addressing the spiritual dimension of care. This recognition of their own limitations indicates that health care professionals still feel uncertain about how to address this aspect of care. This uncertainty may arise because they feel that they do not have sufficient insight or skills to address the spiritual dimension.

Box 6.2 Skills required to provide spiritual care

Good interpersonal and communication skills

Development of trust

Sensitivity

Self-awareness – clarification of personal values

Provision of support to the patient/service users and colleagues

Education and training

Openness and honesty

Multidisciplinary collaboration

Recognition of your own limitations

CAUTION

Caution must be exercised when identifying and discussing the types of skills that health care professionals may require to meet patients' spiritual needs. The danger is to assume that health care professionals do not already possess them. When teaching health care professionals about spiritual care, I conclude my session by stating: 'Many health care professionals already possess many skills required to take the initiative in dealing with patients' spiritual needs. What they sometimes lack is the confidence and education.'

Hierarchy of support

McSherry (2004, p.286–288) identified a hierarchy of support that health care professionals may use to support individuals to meet any spiritual need(s), whether these have been assessed formally or just expressed by the individual. There seemed to be identifiable within the nurses', patients' and the health care professionals' transcripts a 'hierarchy of support'. This hierarchy ranged from providing 'general support', to supporting individuals with 'specific or complex' needs (Figure 6.1). The hierarchy is clearly illustrated in the following transcript:

> Participant (P): 'I actually think that you can help them to achieve their spirituality by sitting (presence) with them, actually and that's okay, if that's what they want? Em, I don't think, it takes any more than that! I think, if you want to listen to them em... [short pause] or if they want to talk (express) about their spirituality, then that's okay, em, but like anything else I might want to talk about it and I might think crumbs, I don't know anything about this, but it's not, about, necessarily about, what they are saying, but it's about your response to it, and the contact or the quality of the contact you have with them... [short pause] does that make sense?' (P 4 Nurse II)

At the base of the pyramid would be the term 'expressing', where individuals feel supported to disclose their worries and concerns, or feel confident to request particular resources. This would move on to the next area of support, that staff are 'receptive and listen' to expressed need. At the middle of the pyramid would be 'presence and facilitation'. Staff are able to provide time and give of themselves to assist patients with requests for help. This may involve the nurse or allied health professional liaising with religious/spiritual leaders or even specialist counsellors, practitioners. Towards the top of the pyramid come religious needs and specialist interventions such as counselling.

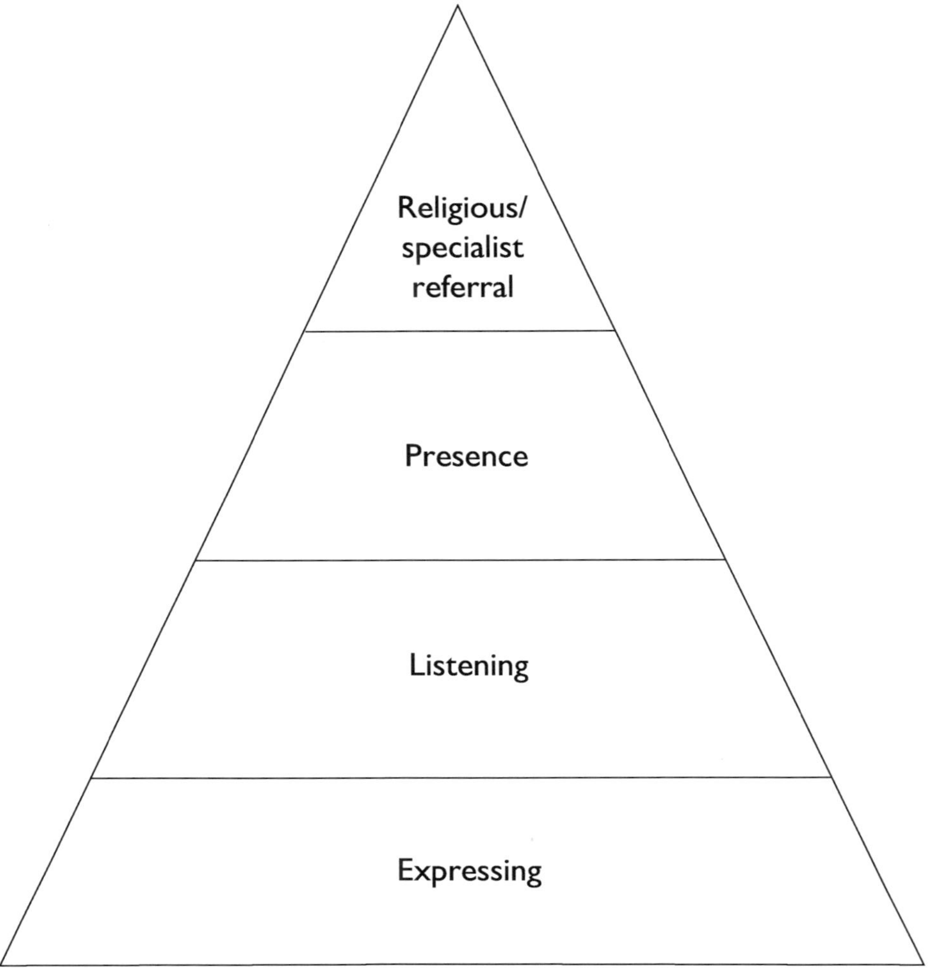

Figure 6.1: Hierarchy of support

The nurses and the health care professionals recognized that there may be certain religious rituals, practices, and emotional, psychological problems that may warrant specialist and continued intervention to help patients to meet specific religious, spiritual needs. The pyramid reveals that spiritual support may be dependent upon several components which, if not present, may inhibit the provision of spiritual care. For example, without the first, 'expressing', the others could not occur.

This hierarchy of support operates at two levels: first, this may be the order in which individual patients test the water for spiritual care. Second, it can be applied to all the allied health professionals in that it describes the types of interventions, the order and sequencing of skills that may need to be used if any form of 'care' including spiritual care is to be provided effectively. This hierarchy can be superimposed on all types of care since spiritual care should be integrated and not fragmented.

Communication/interpersonal skills

It could be argued that communication and interpersonal skills are fundamental to all aspects of health care. This is certainly a central theme in *Essence of Care: Patient-focused Benchmarks for Clinical Governance* (DH 2003), a document aimed at raising standards within health care practice. Without the use of good interpersonal skills and communication, important information may not be conveyed adequately between patient or service user and other health care professionals. Given the deeply sensitive and personal nature of spirituality, there is a greater need for communication to be effective in removing barriers and alleviating fears. It would appear that effective communication is a prerequisite to the formation of any kind of relationship (McCavery 1985). Without the use of good communication, we can never expect to know, understand or become aware of individuals' innermost fears, motives or spiritual concerns.

When addressing an individual's spiritual needs, the health care professional must use all forms of communication and interpersonal skills to identify and evaluate the problem. It is not the intention of this section to explore all aspects of communication, but rather to identify methods that are important when attending to patients' spiritual concerns. Three important aspects of communication that seem pertinent to the issue of spiritual care are attentive listening, non-verbal communication and the use of presence (Box 6.3).

Attentive listening

A brief definition of attentive listening is provided. However, there is more to attentive listening than merely paying attention. We can give all the indications to a patient and service user that we are listening when in reality we hear little about what they have expressed. Burnard (1988a, p.371) warns us of this hidden danger:

> The first practical step in helping others with spiritual problems, then, is listening to them. This may seem so obvious as to not need stating. However we often spend considerable time with others rehearsing our replies to what they are saying, rather than truly listening to them.

Box 6.3 Terms defined

Attentive listening

This means listening to and not necessarily saying anything as the patient discloses his or her spiritual need. It is about paying attention to words, tone of voice and non-verbal language. Attentive listening is not a shallow activity but one that allows you to engage with the patient at a deeper level.

Non-verbal communication

The area of non-verbal communication is crucial in generating a therapeutic relationship between health care professional and patient. Health care professionals must have an insight into the non-verbal gestures, expressions and body language that they display. They must be able to observe the non-verbal cues exhibited by their patients and service users.

Presence, or making time

By far the greatest consolation an individual can have when experiencing a spiritual concern is knowing that someone is there for him or her in this time of need. Presence means being with the individual in a physical, psychological and spiritual sense.

It would appear that attentive listening is about focusing upon what the patient or service user has to say and clearing our head of any judgements, ideas or opinions that we have concerning the problem, thereby giving our undivided attention. In situations that are intense and stressful, there is a tendency for us to fill the silence. However, silence can be a powerful tool in that it allows individuals to think, reflect and process points that may have been raised. When facilitating workshops on spiritual care, it is always tempting to fill natural silences with speech, especially if the content of what was being discussed prior to the silence was emotionally challenging. Morrison (1992) tells us that possibly the best form of communication is silence.

Narayanasamy (1997) provides a list of attributes of a good listener. These are summarized here:

- Generating an environment and counselling relationship in which the patient or service user feels he or she is being listened to.
- Giving your complete attention to the patient or service user. Suspending your own thoughts and opinions on the subject – clearing your own head.
- Using reflection and paraphrasing to indicate you are giving full attention, and listening hard.
- Responding warmly to the patient or service user. Using open gestures and speech to encourage the individual to talk, indicating acceptance of his or her spiritual need.

It must be stressed that attentive listening is difficult. This particular skill is not developed overnight but through much experience and practice. The use of prolonged attentive listening can be demanding, resulting in the health care professional feeling exhausted. This is because such interventions require the nurse to enter into a relationship that draws upon his or her own spiritual reserves. Therefore, attentive listening is not easy because it is time-consuming and demanding. However, the benefits of simply listening to and allowing patients to express their inner concerns, fears and spiritual needs can in itself be therapeutic. As part of listening, the nurse may also be observing for other non-verbal cues that indicate the patient has a spiritual need.

Activity 6.1

Consider the points that have been raised in this section regarding attentive listening. Write down what attributes are to be found in a good listener. Can you think of any ways in which we can improve our listening skills?

Non-verbal communication

The importance of observation was stressed in the section addressing assessment (Chapter 4). An important part of assessment is being alert to factors or cues that may be suggestive of a patient having spiritual need(s). McSherry (1996) recalls how a patient's non-verbal behaviours indicated a deep spiritual need as summarised in Case study 6.2.

Case study 6.2 The importance of non-verbal communication

A patient was withdrawn, used limited communication and detached herself from any form of interaction with other patients. It emerged after several days that the patient had experienced a great loss and needed time to grieve and reconcile, adjusting to the loss. This resulted in her displaying the non-verbal cues that the nurses interpreted as odd. The nurses reacted to the cues in a judgemental manner, viewing the patient's behaviour as antagonistic. The patient was immediately labelled unpopular (Stockwell 1984). (Adapted from McSherry, 1996).

This brief case study illustrates the importance of health care professionals being alert to the unspoken words of patients and service users. It warns us of the danger of attaching the wrong interpretation to different non-verbal behaviours displayed by individuals. If we observe a patient adopting the foetal position because of a severe abdominal pain, we would not dismiss this and say 'it is trapped wind' and provide no analgesia to assist in alleviating the pain and discomfort. A fundamental principle in pain management is you always believe the pain is what the patient tells you. A major principle we need to remember in the management of spiritual pain is never to make value judgements based on our interpretations of non-verbal behaviours. Elsdon (1995, p.642) illustrates this when addressing the concept of spiritual pain:

> The cure for physical pain may be analgesia, but the cure for spiritual pain is to be found in the experience of the pain itself. Spiritual pain, then, is not so much a 'problem to be solved', as a 'question to be lived', and thus demands different qualities in health-care professionals.

We have indicated that communication is a two-way process – an interaction between, for example, the nurse and the patient. There is a need for all health care professionals involved in the provision of spiritual care to be aware of their own non-verbal language. The amount of appropriate eye contact given during an interaction when dealing with a patient presenting with a spiritual need can convey the professional's level of concern and empathy. For example, a consultant who walks into the consulting room to break bad news and is constantly looking at the clock on the wall does not convey empathy or sensitivity to the individual's needs. Likewise, the junior doctor who informs relatives that a loved one has died, while standing with his or her arms folded and backed up against the wall, does not inspire confidence.

When providing spiritual care, a conscious awareness of our non-verbal signals is required. The way in which the health care professional sits can encourage the patient or service user to feel at ease and relaxed. Adopting an open posture (arms and legs not crossed) and sitting in a relaxed manner, leaning slightly towards the individual, will encourage dialogue (Burnard 1988a). It must be stressed that such skills do not develop overnight, and neither do they develop through a process of osmosis in the clinical skills facility, although this can be a useful training ground. Counselling skills only become a natural and spontaneous part of the nurse after considerable use in practice. It is worth remembering that we are all beginners and mistakes will be made (Morrison 1992). However, it is how we reflect and learn from our experiences that is important and developmental.

Developing trust

Patients or service users will not disclose their spiritual needs in an environment that is alien, unfriendly or hostile. In fact, effective spiritual care can only be provided in an environment that is totally the opposite. Individuals need to feel that health care professionals can be trusted with their spiritual needs. Trust will only be established if patients and service users feel that a nurse or any health care professional is both reliable and dependable. When undertaking workshops on spirituality, a question I am frequently asked is 'Why do patients disclose their spiritual needs to you?' After spending many years pondering upon this question, my response is 'Patients feel that they can trust me and that I am dependable and reliable'. Further reflection into why a patient may perceive these qualities in me is because I try to make time for them in meeting simple everyday requests (Box 6.4). The illustration in Box 6.4 may be verging on the ridiculous, but this approach is what I feel encourages patients to disclose personal and sensitive needs to me.

Interestingly, while conducting interviews for my PhD studies, a patient whom I interviewed said the following, confirming my thoughts that, if patients or service users feel that they can trust us with something that seems insignificant, then they will feel that they can trust and relate to us with much more important matters:

> Participant (P) 'You get care in hospice because you are important to them and there are fewer numbers. In a hospital you are getting medical treatment plus a bit of food. I say, if you say to somebody, hey nurse I haven't got me glasses can you bring me, how about a glass of water, I'll bring you one.' (P 14 Patient I)

> The patient went on to say that in the hospice he would have a glass of water provided before he even asked. (McSherry 2004, pp.246–247)

Narayanasamy (1997, p.215) confirms this: 'Trust grows over a period of time as the client tests the environment, risks self-disclosure, and observes the carer's adherence to commitment.'

Box 6.4 A simple illustration

A patient asks you for a jug of water. You are busy because of staff shortages. Your immediate response to the patient is 'I will be back in a minute'. The nurse's minute must be the longest minute on earth. Perhaps several hours later you remember the patient's request, but by then it is too late and someone else has satisfied his or her thirst. My response to such a request is to fetch the water immediately, if I am not undertaking a task of greater priority. The patient is satisfied and forms an impression of you based on reliability and dependability. If patients feel that they can trust you in simple matters, like filling a jug of water, then they will trust you in matters of greater importance.

Patients and service users are not passive recipients of care: they are constantly assessing the situation and undertaking a personal audit of the skills and services available in a particular area. They assess the qualities that individual members of staff display (obviously this process is not undertaken if the patient is unconscious or has a cognitive impairment), reaching an opinion based on their own judgements and expectations. This is a possible reason why certain health care professionals or members of staff are used frequently by patients or service users to disclose their innermost concerns. Trust-building is a skill that can be developed by all health care professionals. It only takes a minute to sow the seeds of trust and respect. Trust can be developed by utilizing the other skills addressed in previous sections.

Sensitivity

Spiritual care cannot be provided if the health care professional is not sensitive to the needs of individual patients and service users. Spirituality has been explored within the context of holism (Chapter 3). This discussion demonstrated that we are all unique individuals made up of many interactive systems, which are constantly changing and developing according to environmental, political, social and economic forces. Therefore, individuals and their spirituality are constantly changing and evolving – adapting to different circumstances, both positive and negative, across the lifespan. It is highly unlikely, then, that a health care professional will encounter two patients or service users with exactly the same spiritual need.

A health care professional may have to address spiritual needs stemming from deep-rooted conflict, unresolved anger, frustration or guilt. All these may have affected the individual's system for months or years. Such spiritual needs must be handled in a sensitive manner without judgement being passed (Case study 4.6). Likewise, the health care professional may have to support patients and service users who have been diagnosed with a terminal disease, helping them prepare for death (Elsdon 1995; Schoenbeck 1994).

For some individuals, their spirituality may be shaped and expressed through formal religious affiliation and worship. Health care professionals may have to assist individuals in maintaining their religious practices while in receipt of health care. Religion is a very sensitive subject that can arouse strong emotions. Some individuals – health care professional, patient or service user – can become very protective of their own personal beliefs if they feel these are being challenged or brought into question. Therefore, all health care professionals must deal with matters of religion sensitively. Perhaps what makes matters of religion difficult to address is that they can challenge our own personal beliefs and values about the meaning of life and existence (Burnard 1988a).

Read Case study 6.3 and write down any areas that you feel would require sensitive handling.

Case study 6.3 A need for sensitivity

Victoria is admitted to your ward with a suspected drug overdose of heroin. She is a single parent, having three young children by three different fathers. Victoria earns money by working as a prostitute in the city. The medical team stabilizes Victoria's condition and after several days in hospital she makes a full recovery. In the meantime, her children have been fostered out to other families by social services. Victoria is annoyed and frustrated at the interventions by social services and is concerned that her children will not be returned to her because this is her third suicide attempt within three months.

The case study contains several issues – addiction, prostitution, overdose, fostering of children – that if not dealt with sensitively could turn the situation into a confrontation. It is evident that Victoria is experiencing a great deal of turbulence in her life and is searching for support and meaning. The biggest danger is that some health care professionals may make a judgement based on her heroin addiction and her prostitution – viewing her as a loser. Such an evaluation would be unsafe and unfair because we are not aware of all the variables in the equation that may have resulted in Victoria taking the path into drugs and prostitution. The correct way of addressing this situation is to ensure that Victoria receives the same spiritual care as any other patient on the ward. We should be making no distinctions based on her lifestyle or history. The case study highlights that, if health care professionals are to be successful in this challenge, then they need to be in touch with their own personal beliefs and values (Burnard 1988a; Harrison 1993; Narayanasamy 1997).

Honesty

No communication will be effective if a relationship is not based upon honesty and trust. The area of spiritual care is no exception – it requires the health care professional delivering spiritual care to be honest and open. If a patient or service user finds that individuals have not been open and honest about aspects of care and diagnosis and the truth is eventually revealed, then the individual concerned can be left feeling hurt and alone, adding further to a dispirited state. McCavery (1985, p.140) writes:

> It is difficult to imagine any aspect of nursing where truth is more important than in the area of spiritual care. Yet half-truths, or even lies, are often commonplace in respect of patients with poor prognosis. Phrases such as 'Of course you're going to get better', or 'Don't be worried, you'll be home in no time', come from professionals and relatives alike.

Read Case study 6.4 and write down how you might have handled this situation. Pay particular attention to possible reasons why health care professionals and family may find it difficult to tell the truth.

One reason why health care professionals may not want to tell the truth is fear of causing distress to the patient or service user. By dressing up bad news in ambiguous language, it protects the individual from the full force of reality. An example of this is saying, 'You have a growth'. This also shields the health care professional, acting as a defence mechanism. These factors may be operating in Case study 6.4. Frank's family are trying to protect him from the reality of the situation by seeking alternative ways of addressing the question

Case study 6.4 To tell or not to tell?

Frank, aged 65, is rushed to the ward following resuscitation in the outpatient department. On admission to your ward, Frank is semiconscious and the medical staff feel death is imminent. Frank's next of kin are notified and asked to come into the ward. However, the medical staff's prediction is proved wrong and several days later Frank is still alive, floating in and out of consciousness. The medical staff believe that Frank's present condition is the result of an abdominal tumour. One afternoon while on duty, you notice that Frank's relative is a little anxious and concerned. Upon enquiry, the relative reveals that Frank is a practising Roman Catholic and the relative would like his priest to come and administer the sacrament of the sick. However, the relative is aware that Frank, despite his strong faith, is still fearful of death. The relative is also unsure about whether to tell Frank about his diagnosis and prognosis.

How might you address this situation?

of his anticipated death. Certainly they do not want to cause him any distress, given his current condition. However, the chances are that Frank is very much aware of his situation. This form of deception can destroy trust, especially if an individual suspects that things are not what they seem and insists on answers. When the individual is made aware of the correct diagnosis, he or she can feel angry and hurt, even betrayed. It is difficult for nurses because they are often arbitrators with limited power, having to respect the authority of the consultant while acting as advocate for the patient. However, this relationship is changing and nurses are often present when bad news is given and in some areas of work nurses actually take the lead in this area.

Increasingly, some areas of health care practice now have advocacy systems or patient advocates who support patient and service users through the difficulties they encounter in health care.

The old maxim 'honesty is the best policy' certainly applies when addressing spiritual needs. Looking at Case study 6.4, how might you address this situation? You could contact the Roman Catholic chaplain and ask him to do a general visit to the ward. This approach may not distress Frank, who may think that the priest visits the ward as a matter of course. Alternatively, you might consult Frank when conscious and ask him what he wants and what he feels. This latter approach would do more to promote trust and honesty – especially if Frank were to recover.

Self-awareness

Self-awareness is fundamental to the fostering of relationships that will prove effective in meeting patients' spiritual needs. Several authors (Burnard 1988a; Harrison 1993; Narayanasamy 1997) underline the importance of developing personal awareness of one's own beliefs and values when providing spiritual care. McSherry (1996, p.49) writes: 'Spiritual awareness does not imply religiosity or piety, but the ability to explore positively one's own attitudes and feelings about matters that are fundamental to our existence.'

The quotation indicates that there is a need for all nurses and indeed people working within health care to have insight or self-awareness of their own beliefs and values. Self-awareness or personal value clarification is not just for the religious but is applicable to all health care professionals. Like many of the other skills mentioned in this chapter, self-awareness requires nurturing and developing. Our self-awareness can change as our values, beliefs or attitudes change through exposure to different situations or events that may occur in life or practice. Self-awareness can be developed through training. Self-awareness concerns the development and acknowledgement of our own inner thoughts, feelings and behaviours. This insight is important if we are to accept and understand ourselves. Without this personal understanding and insight we are probably less likely to be able to understand others (Burnard 1988a; Narayanasamy 1997; Ross 1997). By fostering our own spiritual awareness we will be more focused and receptive to those who may have a spiritual concern (Elsdon 1995; Schoenbeck 1994). Ross (1997, p.167) identified the association between self-awareness and the delivery of spiritual care:

> Firstly, concerning the nurse, it seemed that nurses who demonstrated a personal search for meaning in their own lives, although they identified a narrow range of spiritual needs, gave spiritual care at a deeper level than those who did not demonstrate this characteristic.

Ross' conclusions reinforce the need for nurses and indeed all health care professionals to develop self-awareness or else the type of spiritual care provided may not go beyond superficial enquiry into religious affiliation (although necessary), which does not constitute spiritual care at a deeper level.

Three methods that can be used to generate self-awareness are reflection, critical analysis and appraisal of oneself and experiences (Figure 6.2). Reflection is normally a retrospective activity – thinking about the event or incident

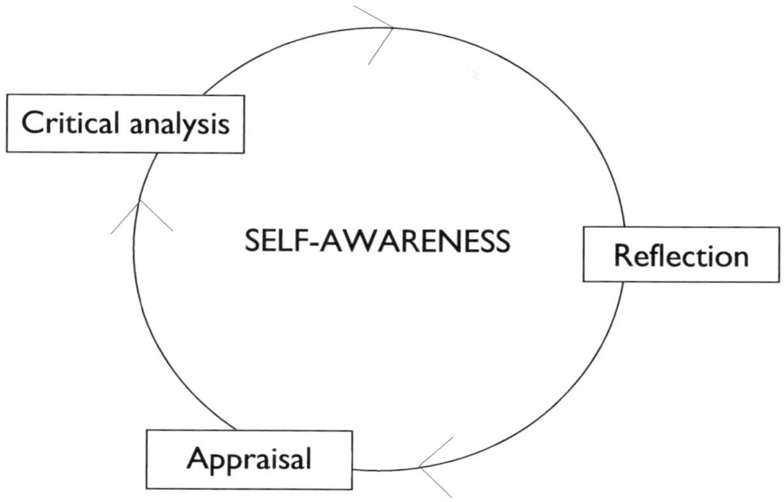

Figure 6.2: Methods that can develop self-awareness

after it has passed. Reflection is about reviewing a situation, questioning one's thoughts, feelings or personal actions. We can all reflect upon situations but we may not act upon what we have learned or discovered. Critical analysis is looking at a situation in more detail. It is not merely reflecting upon the situation but implies reviewing and considering all aspects in a balanced manner. Critical appraisal is more in-depth and structured than reflection. Appraisal is usually performed by a third party. We may ask a colleague to observe our actions or responses in a particular situation and provide verbal or written feedback. These three methods provide us with an insight into our behaviours, feelings and attitudes. If we use one in isolation from the rest, we may only become aware of ourselves in monochrome. If we use two methods, we may see more detail and the picture will be in colour. By employing all three methods, we build up a '3D' picture of ourselves, our emotions and our feelings and in this way become self-aware.

However, one fundamental ingredient is required in utilizing any of these methods – time alone. We can only truly find and understand ourselves by going into our own inner wilderness. We cannot find ourselves in the constant bustle of modern living. Solitude and stillness are necessary if the individual is to enter into a dialogue with self. This is evident in the writings of many religious or spiritual leaders who, in order to find themselves, physically withdrew from the world, isolating themselves from material distractions. Obviously this method is not being advocated. However, the principle of spending time alone for five minutes a day reflecting, critically analysing situations or questioning our actions to a particular patient/service user or event will develop self-awareness.

There are other methods that can be helpful in developing self-awareness. Harrison and Burnard (1993) advocate the use of a 'Spiritual values clarification questionnaire', which can be completed by individuals undertaking workshops on spirituality. The questionnaire encourages the individual to focus upon self, questioning personal beliefs, values and attitudes towards spirituality. The questionnaire is a useful activity for encouraging debate and dialogue.

In summary, self-awareness is essential to our own spiritual and personal growth. It would be a grave error to assume that only the methods mentioned in this section can develop self-awareness. There are many different exercises that can lead to individuals developing self-awareness. Once aware of the need for self-awareness, many people use methods or exercises that suit their own personalities and social circumstances.

Activity 6.2

Spend five minutes, alone, in a quiet place reflecting upon an event or incident that involved you. Ask yourself several questions – How did I feel at the time? How do I feel now? Why did I feel that way? Could I have reacted any differently? What would I change if the situation reoccurred? What have I learned about myself and others?

Support

By now you will have realized that the provision of spiritual care is not easy in that it can be emotionally and spiritually draining for all involved. It is important to recognize that we are not alone in the provision of spiritual care. There is a need for support from colleagues and other health care professionals with whom we work (Burnard 1988a). Counselling can be very demanding and individuals may find that they do not have sufficient skills or resources to address a patient's or service user's particular need. Sometimes a health care professional and patient/service user may have grown too close so that judgements are clouded or obscured. In such situations, the health care professional and the patient/service user may require support from colleagues to work through the situation.

Collaboration

It is correct to state that no single professional group has the monopoly in relation to the provision of spiritual care (Stoter 1995). However, it must be recognized that nurses are in a unique position in that the nature of their work and their duty rostering means that they have contact with patients 24 hours a day, 7 days a week and 52 weeks a year. Stoter (1995, p.137) emphasizes the unique and central role that the nurse plays as the facilitator of spiritual care:

> It is important to make the point here that the prime responsibility for giving continuous spiritual care inevitably lies with the nursing staff who are there all the time. They are likely to be the key people, if not always, for the in-depth care at least as facilitators of that process with the responsibility to ensure that spiritual care is given.

However, this still does not mean that nurses are solely responsible for providing spiritual care. In fact, research suggests nurses feel that a multidisciplinary approach is required if patients' spiritual needs are to be met (Keighley 1997; McSherry 1997; Narayanasamy 1993; Waugh 1992).

McSherry's (1997) results confirm that nurses do not perceive themselves as the main providers of spiritual care. Of the 549 nurses surveyed, 76.7 per cent (421) felt that spiritual care should be provided by a combination of people. This combination included nurses, chaplains, patient, family, friends and the patient's own religious leader. The overwhelming response to this question indicates that the provision of spiritual care must be flexible and collaborative in that there must be an exchange of information in relation to spiritual care among all parties concerned.

Stoter (1995) urges caution, indicating that at the end of the day it is the patient or his or her relatives who will choose the key person in the delivery of spiritual care. It therefore appears that spiritual care should be managed through teamwork. A team approach to the management of spiritual care will ensure that everyone is working towards the same goal and outcome. However, it would appear that the nurse has a central role to play not only in the identification of such needs, but also in the facilitation of spiritual care. McSherry (2004) found that inter- and intra-disciplinary team working was paramount in supporting individuals presenting with a spiritual/religious need. Furthermore, the research suggests that patients and service users will identify their own 'spiritual resource' person; this could be a volunteer working in the practice area or indeed the consultant or chaplain. This finding stresses the importance of good communication and inter-professional collaboration.

Religious needs

Through collaboration and liaising with chaplains, patients or service users who have a spiritual need(s) that stems from their affiliation with a formal religion can access support. Through collaboration, such individuals will receive expert advice and support. There may be occasions when a patient or service user asks a health care professional about a matter of theology or religious doctrine that they are unable to address. In such instances, they should and can enlist the services of the hospital chaplain or the patient's own spiritual/religious leader.

Box 6.5 Reflection on chaplaincy

Orchard (2001, p.13) outlines that there is a diminishing debate about the professional status of chaplaincy. This debate is still rumbling concerning the central place that chaplains have within the multidisciplinary team. Cobb (2001) suggests that this debate is associated with the moral basis of chaplaincy implying that this needs to be more rigorous. This debate is extremely complex and I do not want to play down the fundamental issues debated. However, it is my own personal opinion that failure to give chaplaincy full recognition within the health care team will be detrimental to health care. Chaplains in some areas are not accepted as health care professionals, meaning they do not have the same rights of access to information as other groups. I certainly do not agree with this argument and feel that this is a major limitation to service delivery and organization. The government and the Department of Health need to address this matter with some urgency so that these issues are resolved giving chaplaincy equal rights and standing to all the other health care professions.

Health care professionals need to be aware that the chaplain has a specific pastoral function to play. Chaplains are there not only to support patients or service users in their time of need, but are also a valuable source of support to other health care workers. Many chaplains within National Health Service and Primary Care Trusts are now termed 'ecumenical', or 'generic' in that they provide support to all religious denominations and are only too willing to offer support (Elsdon 1995; Leggieri 1986; Speck 1992).

Danger of proselytising

With respect to the provision of spiritual care, health care professionals need to protect patients and service users from religious zealots and sects who seek to convert vulnerable people. Health care professionals need to be on their guard against organizations that may access health care institutions with a view to converting or preaching to individuals who have no means of escape. Many Trusts do not allow organizations access unless they have sought the appropriate approval. However, some do slip through the net and all health care professionals must be vigilant.

The non-believer

Another area that must be considered under this section of religious needs is the spiritual needs of the non-believer. Health care professionals must also address the spiritual needs of the atheist and agnostic. Assuming that spiritual care is only relevant to those who have a strong religious faith is misguided. Atheists and agnostics may still raise existential questions and be in need of spiritual care (Burnard 1988b; Narayanasamy 2001). It is on such occasions that the health care professionals must provide care that is appropriate. Arranging a visit from the hospital chaplain could be perceived as offensive (McSherry 1996). The health care team will need to support such patients or service users without the involvement of any religious organization.

Recognition of our own limitations

One of the gravest mistakes any health care professional can make in supporting individuals with spiritual needs is not to acknowledge their limitations and therefore work outside their level of competency. To continue in an interaction with a patient or service user that is beyond one's level of expertise or control is dangerous and potentially damaging. If a health care professional feels that a situation has entered a different or difficult phase that is beyond his or her level of expertise, then this should be recognized and discussed between both parties involved. It is unrealistic to imagine that we have answers or solutions to every spiritual need that will be encountered – given the unique and personal nature of spirituality.

The health care professional must therefore acknowledge this and be prepared to say to patients or service users:

> I am sorry but I have not got any answers to this question.

or

> I can see that you still require support in this matter. However, I feel that I cannot help you any further but I can refer you on to someone who has a little more knowledge in this area.

This public acceptance of one's own limitations in no way constitutes failure. Carson (1989) and Harrison (1993) feel that this public acknowledgement constitutes humility, which is an essential element for personal spiritual growth.

Some authors have argued that health care professionals may not possess the skills to adequately address patients who are experiencing spiritual needs. Burnard (1988a) and Harrison (1993) feel that for the spiritually distressed patient or service user basic counselling skills are not enough. While this appears to be a criticism of the practitioners' abilities, the point does warrant further explanation. Burnard and Harrison are not being critical but making a valid observation in that, although some health care professionals and specifically nurses do possess some basic counselling skills, these may not be sufficient to help individuals with deep-rooted problems. Such individuals may require the release of emotions that will require regular contact with a counsellor over an extended period of time. Therefore, health care professionals need to assess the full situation before entering into a counselling relationship with patients or service users who have spiritual needs. Conversely, Burnard and Harrison's observation does not act as an 'opt out' clause since they are alerting nurses and health care professionals to the hidden traps, not stating that health care professionals should not provide spiritual care.

Conclusion

This chapter has introduced you to some of the fundamental skills necessary for the provision of spiritual care. However, it has been suggested that it is often difficult to differentiate between essential care and spiritual care. The chapter indicates that health care professionals may already possess many of the skills necessary to provide spiritual care and what they sometimes lack is confidence in the application of such skills to the spiritual dimension. The chapter suggests that the entire area of spiritual care requires commitment from the health care professional and the organizations/institutions, and that addressing spiritual needs of patients or service users will be demanding and spiritually exhausting. The importance of having self-awareness to better meet patients' and service users' spiritual needs has been stressed. It has been indicated that health care professionals will only become proficient in attending to patients' or service users' spiritual needs if they take a risk and become involved. By providing spiritual care, health care professionals may also attain deeper insights into their own spirituality.

References

Burnard, P. (1987) 'Spiritual distress and the nursing response: theoretical considerations and counselling skills.' *Journal of Advanced Nursing 12*, 377–382.

Burnard, P. (1988a) 'Discussing spiritual issues with clients.' *Health Visitor 61* (December) 371–372.

Burnard, P. (1988b) 'The spiritual needs of atheists and agnostics.' *Professional Nurse* (December) 130–132.

Carson, V.B. (1989) *Spiritual Dimensions of Nursing Practice.* Philadelphia: WB Saunders.

Cobb, M. (2001) 'Walking on water? The moral foundations of chaplaincy.' In H. Orchard (ed.) (2001) *Spirituality in Health Care Contexts*, 73–83. London: Jessica Kingsley Publishers.

Department of Health (DH) (2003) *Essence of Care: Patient-focused Benchmarking for Clinical Governance.* London: Department of Health.

Elsdon, M. (1995) 'Spiritual pain in dying people: the nurse's role.' *Professional Nurse 10*, 10, 641–643.

Harrison, J. (1993) 'Spirituality and nursing practice.' *Journal of Clinical Nursing 2*, 211–217.

Harrison, J. and Burnard, P. (1993) *Spirituality and Nursing Practice.* Aldershot: Avebury.

Keighley, T. (1997) 'Organizational structures and personal spiritual belief.' *International Journal of Palliative Nursing 3*, 1, 47–51.

Leggieri, J. (1986) 'Pastoral care in hospital: uniqueness and contribution.' *Topics in Clinical Nursing 8*, 2, 47–55.

McCavery, R. (1985) 'Spiritual care in acute illness.' In O. McGilloway and F. Myco (eds) *Nursing and Spiritual Care.* London: Harper and Row.

McSherry, W. (1996) 'Raising the spirits.' *Nursing Times 92*, 3, 48–49.

McSherry, W. (1997) 'A descriptive survey of nurses' perceptions of spirituality and spiritual care.' Unpublished MPhil thesis, Hull: University of Hull.

McSherry, W. (2004) 'The meaning of spirituality and spiritual care: an investigation of health care professionals', patients' and public's perceptions.' Unpublished PhD thesis. Leeds: Leeds Metropolitan University.

Morrison, R. (1992) 'Diagnosing pain in patients.' *Nursing Standard 11*, 6, 36–38.

Narayanasamy, A. (1993) 'Nurses' awareness and educational preparation in meeting their patients' spiritual needs.' *Nurse Education Today 13*, 3, 196–201.

Narayanasamy, A. (1997) 'Spiritual dimensions of learning disability.' In B. Gates and C. Beacock (eds) *Dimensions of Learning Disability*, 203–222. London: Baillière Tindall.

Narayanasamy, A. (2001) *Spiritual Care: A Practical Guide for Nurses and Health Care Practitioners*, 2nd edn. Wiltshire: Quay Publishing.

Orchard, H. (ed.) (2001) *Spirituality in Health Care: Contexts.* London: Jessica Kingsley Publishers.

Ross, L.A. (1997) *Nurses' Perceptions of Spiritual Care. Developments in Nursing and Health Care 13.* Aldershot: Avebury.

Schoenbeck, S.L. (1994) 'Called to care: addressing the spiritual needs of patients.' *Journal of Practical Nursing* (September) 19–23.

Speck, P. (1992) 'Nursing the soul.' *Nursing Times 88*, 23, 22.

Stockwell, F. (1984) *The Unpopular Patient.* London: Croom Helm.

Stoter, D. (1995) *Spiritual Aspects of Health Care.* London: Mosby.

Waugh, L.A. (1992) 'Spiritual aspects of nursing: a descriptive study of nurses' perceptions.' Unpublished PhD thesis, Edinburgh: Queen Margaret College.

Further reading

Many books have been written on the subject of counselling and communication skills in nursing and health care and such books may have been recommended as part of a course. With respect to counselling, you are advised to consult any of these texts. The articles and books listed below will consolidate some of the issues that have been raised in the chapter. Although some of the references may appear dated, the work of these authors is still relevant and appropriate.

Burnard, P. (1987) 'Spiritual distress and the nursing response: theoretical considerations and counselling skills.' *Journal of Advanced Nursing 12*, 377–382.

Burnard, P. (1988) 'Discussing spiritual issues with clients.' *Health Visitor 61* (December), 371– 372.

Jenkins, B. (2002) 'Offering spiritual care.' In B. Rumbold (2002) *Spirituality and Palliative Care*, 116–129. Australia: Oxford University Press.

Johnson, A. (1998) 'The notion of spiritual care in professional practice.' In M. Cobb and V. Robshaw *The Spiritual Challenge of Health Care*, 151–166. Edinburgh: Churchill Livingstone.

Robinson, S., Kendrick, K. and Brown, B. (2003) *Spirituality and the Practice of Health Care*, 92–120. Houndmill: Palgrave Macmillan.

Stoter, D. (1995) *Spiritual Aspects of Health Care.* London: Mosby.

CHAPTER 7

Developments in Spirituality

Research and Education

Introduction

Earlier chapters encouraged you to explore the concept of spirituality and the provision of spiritual care with the intention of generating self-awareness. In this chapter, we will undertake a brief review of some pioneering research that has been conducted concerning spirituality and spiritual health care. The research studies presented address both health care professionals' and patients' perceptions of the spiritual dimension. By reading this chapter you should gain a richer and fuller understanding of how the spiritual dimension is being perceived and developed within health care practice and education. By critically analysing and reflecting upon the studies you will build on your previous reflections, developing a deeper insight into the terms spirituality and spiritual care as perceived by health care professionals, patients and service users. The emerging educational debate surrounding spirituality and education is introduced at the end of this chapter.

Activity 7.1

Before proceeding further with this chapter, write down anything that you know and understand about the term research. You may want to consider which approach to research is used most frequently in your discipline – for example, qualitative or quantitative.

In your reflections, you have possibly written down a great deal of information concerning your understanding of the term research. The amount of knowledge and insight that you have into research may be dependent upon how much education you received on the subject during your programme of education. The glossary of terms provided (Box 7.1) is designed to give a basic insight so that you can appraise some of the studies that have been undertaken by researchers into the spiritual dimension.

Box 7.1 A brief overview of some of the most common terminology used in research

Qualitative

Research that addresses concepts that are very personal and subjective, such as individuals' feelings, thoughts and values.

Quantitative

Research that is scientific and systematic, generating numerical figures for analysis.

Research process

A term used to describe the different stages involved in undertaking a research study.

Validity

Research is said to be valid if it actually achieves the results that it set out to achieve, or an instrument measures what it is supposed to measure.

Reliability

That a piece of research or instrument can consistently measure or be repeated over time.

Evidence-based care

Now a frequently used term that implies that health care professionals use the most up-to-date research findings to inform nursing practice.

Data

The information gained while undertaking a piece of research. There are different types of data dependent upon the type of research undertaken – numerical and descriptive.

For further information on any aspect of research, you are encouraged to consult one of the many texts that have been written on the subject (see the Further Reading list at the end of the chapter).

Studies investigating spirituality and spiritual care

A review of the literature suggests that there has been a tremendous number of research studies conducted investigating health care professionals' perceptions of spirituality and spiritual care. Most of the studies undertaken appear to investigate patients' perspectives, with primarily the nurses or other health care professional as an adjunct – for example, see Conrad 1985; Dunn 1993; Emblen and Halstead 1993; Highfield 1992. However, since the publication of the first edition of this book, there has been a noticeable increase in the number of international studies that have focused upon a range of issues associated with spiritual health care. Interestingly, most health care professions are now contributing to this growing body of evidence. A summary of some of these studies is provided in Table 7.1. The research undertaken in this very important area raises questions about how health care professionals interpret and provide spiritual care. The following section presents some of the research findings addressing spirituality and spiritual care. The studies are presented in chronological order and the contribution and the importance of the research findings are explored.

CAUTION

I am very much aware that research into the spiritual dimension is ongoing. The research studies presented in this chapter are by no means comprehensive critiques, nor are they exhaustive in that they represent all research undertaken at a given point in time. The purpose of presenting these studies is to demonstrate how the spiritual dimension has been addressed both theoretically and clinically during the last decade. The author has been selective in the studies presented. It must be emphasized that interest in the spiritual dimension is growing with the majority of health care professionals contributing to the emerging body of knowledge. Therefore, to reiterate, the research presented within this chapter is not representative of all research undertaken or completed within health care addressing the spiritual dimension.

As part of my PhD studies (McSherry 2004), I undertook a literature review and identified 23 international studies (Table 7.1) that utilized qualitative methodologies (for example, phenomenology, ethnography, grounded theory) with eight originating from within the UK. In terms of quantitative studies only, 10 international studies (13 including the three studies that had used multiple methods) were identified. Perhaps one explanation for this disparity in research methods between qualitative and quantitative stems from the deeply subjective and personal nature of spirituality. The personal nature of spirituality means some form of rapport must exist between the researcher and the participant. This can be hard to achieve in several forms of quantitative research – for example, survey methods that employ questionnaires. The following section originates from my thesis (McSherry 2004, pp.109–117).

I hope readers will find this section a useful starting point for reviewing the empirical literature on spirituality.

Activity 7.2

If you have access to electronic databases such as CINHAL, MEDLINE or some that are specific to your own professional group, type in the words 'spirituality' or 'spiritual care' and review the results. Ask yourself what the results suggest about this aspect of health care.

Central themes identifiable within the empirical literature

Identifiable within the empirical literature are two central themes. The first theme is linked with perceptions of spirituality and spiritual care, while the second theme surrounds the enhancement of spiritual care practices, primarily for patients or service users.

Table 7.1 Selected summary of studies conducted by health care professionals into the spiritual dimension

Studies	Country of origin	Type	Sample size	Sample	Area of focus
Burkhardt (1991, 1994*)	US	**	12	Appalachia women	Describing spirituality
Reed (1991)	US	***	300	100 hospitalized adults with incurable cancer 100 hospitalized adults with no serious illness and 100 well non-hospitalized adults	Determine terminally ill and non-terminally ill patients' preferences for spirituality related interventions
Highfield (1992)	US	***	50	27 nurses 23 patients with primary lung cancer	Spiritual health of oncology patients and how well nurses assess spiritual health
Waugh (1992)	UK	**	793	Qualified nurses	Perceptions of spirituality
Harrison and Burnard (1993)	UK	**	10	Qualified nurses	Understanding spirituality
Narayanasamy (1993)	UK	***	33	Registered nurses	Educational preparedness to meet patients' spiritual needs
Emblen and Halstead (1993)	US	**	38	7 chaplains 19 surgical patients 12 nurses	Defining spiritual needs and interventions
Kearney (1994)	UK	**	11	Patients with MS	Spiritual coping

Table 7.1 *cont.*

Studies	Country of origin	Type	Sample size	Sample	Area of focus
Taylor *et al.* (1994, 1995)	US	***	181	Cancer nurse clinicians	Attitudes, beliefs and definitions of spiritual care
Harrington (1995)	Australia	**	10	Registered nurses	Perceptions of spirituality
Clark and Heidenreich (1995)	US	**	63	Critical care patients	Nursing interventions
Conco (1995)	US	**	10	Christian volunteers	Christian patients' views of spiritual care
Ross (1997)	UK	**	10	Elderly patients	Understanding spirituality
McSherry (1997, 2002*)	UK	***	559	Qualified and unqualified nurses	Perceptions of spirituality
Walton (1997, 1999*)	US	**	13	Myocardial patients	What spirituality means
Thomas and Retsas (1999)	Australia	**	19	Terminal cancer	Spiritual meanings people with terminal cancer give to life experiences
Cavendish *et al.* (2000)	US	**	12	Well adults	Spiritual factors/growth
Walton and St Clair (2000)	US	**	11	Received a cardiac transplant	What spirituality means to heart transplant patients
Carroll (2001)	UK	**	15	Hospice nurses	Exploration of the nature of spirituality and spiritual care

Chiu (2001)	US	**	15	Chinese immigrants with breast cancer	Spiritual resources
Wright (2001)	UK	***	151 Hospices 194 Trusts	Senior chaplains	Features of spiritual care
Hermann (2001)	US	**	19	Hospice patients	Identify dying patients' definitions of spirituality and their spiritual needs
Kuuppelomaki (2001)	Finland	***	328	Nurses working in-patient wards	Spiritual support for terminally ill patients
Narayanasamy and Owens (2001)	UK	**	115	Post-registration nurses	Response to spiritual needs of patients
Daalemann *et al.* (2001)	US	**	35	17 women diabetic patients Type 2 18 women with no self-identified illness	Patient-reported, health-related spirituality
Stranahan (2001)	US	***	102	Nurse practitioners	Spiritual perceptions and attitudes about spiritual care/practices
Strang and Strang (2001)	Sweden	**	20 16 next of kin	Brain tumour patients	Spiritual thoughts and coping
Shirahama and Inoue (2001)	Japan	**	10	People living in a farming community	Explore the concept of spirituality

Continued on next page

Table 7.1 *cont.*

Studies	Country of origin	Type	Sample size	Sample	Area of focus
Tuck *et al.* (2001)	US	***	52	Males living with human immunodeficiency virus (HIV)	Relationship between spirituality and psychosocial factors
Arnold *et al.* (2002)	US	****	47	Opioid-dependent patients	Determine how spirituality is defined
Wright (2002)	UK	**	16 not stated	Key stakeholders in palliative care	Spiritual essence of palliative care
Baldacchino (2002*)	UK	****	70	Myocardial infarction patients	Spiritual coping strategies
O'Driscoll (2002)	UK	***	463	Nurses	Perceptions of spirituality
Narayanasamy *et al.* (2002)	UK	**	10	Learning disability nurses	Meeting spiritual needs of clients
Narayanasamy (2002)	UK	**	15	Chronically ill patients	Spiritual coping mechanisms
Taylor (2003)	US	**	28	Patients with cancer and primary family carergivers	Determine what patients, primary family caregivers expect from nurses regarding the meeting of spiritual needs
Taylor and Mariner (2005)	US	***	224	Adult cancer patients and primary caregivers	Clients' preferences for receiving spiritual care from nurses

* Refers to a paper published from the original dissertation/thesis
** Qualitative
*** Quantitative
**** Multiple methods

Perceptions of spirituality and spiritual care

The quantitative and qualitative studies reviewed appear to focus predominately upon specific groups' perceptions of spirituality. The word 'perception' is used as an umbrella covering words such as beliefs, attitudes and understandings of spirituality. For example, within the UK, Waugh (1992), Harrison and Burnard (1993), McSherry (1997) and, more recently, O'Driscoll (2002) have examined nurses' perceptions of spirituality and spiritual care working predominantly within the National Health Service. The findings of these investigations validate that spirituality is perceived as a universal, multifaceted phenomenon. The findings also reveal that nurses are prepared to be involved in the provision of spiritual care. However, not all nurses felt that they were able to meet their patients' spiritual needs satisfactorily. Other researchers have concentrated on the perceptions of service users – for example, Hermann (2001) interviewed dying patients about their understanding of spirituality, while Kearney (1994), and latterly Strang and Strang (2001), discussed issues of spirituality with patients living with neurological disorders such as multiple sclerosis or brain tumours. These investigations demonstrate that some patients may have difficulty in articulating what constitutes spirituality. However, the studies reveal that patients were prepared to talk about their spiritual beliefs, identifying spirituality as an important factor in helping them cope with their illness, or impending death.

Activity 7.3

In your experience, do you think that if you asked patients the question 'Do you have any spiritual needs?' they would understand what you were asking?

Another positive benefit of the research investigating perceptions of spirituality and spiritual care is that some of the studies have led to the development of several scales that assist researchers to measure aspects of the spiritual dimension – for example, the Spiritual Well Being Scale (SWB) (Paloutzain and Ellison 1979), the Spirituality and Spiritual Care Rating Scale (SSCRS) (McSherry 1997; McSherry, Draper and Kendrick 2002), the Spiritual Assessment Inventory (SAI) (Hall and Edwards 2002) and the Spiritual Coping Strategies Scale (SCS) (Baldacchino 2002; Baldacchino and Buhagiar 2003). These instruments have been used successfully in a variety of situations with diverse groups of individuals, and provide valuable insights into how individuals perceive spirituality and how spirituality can be a powerful force in coping with illness and disease.

Activity 7.4

Consider the points that have been raised in this book regarding the assessment of spiritual needs. Why do you think health care professionals may have difficulty in undertaking such assessments? And why is it hard to measure health care professionals' ability to identify patients' spiritual needs?

Additionally, research that targets the spiritual care practices of specialist practitioners has been undertaken – for example, Taylor, Highfield and Amenta (1994) used a questionnaire to determine what spiritual care practices oncology nurses used in their dealings with patients. Frequent practices identified in this investigation were praying with patients, referring to chaplains, and use of presence as well as listening and talking to patients. Taylor *et al.* (1994) were concerned with the findings because a question mark was raised about the nurses' commitment to, or confidence in, providing spiritual care, suggesting that this was not as strong as it could be.

Stranahan (2001) examined the spiritual perceptions and practices among nurse practitioners working in a range of clinical situations; interestingly, the term nurse practitioner was not defined. This is important because the term practitioner can have many meanings, given the proliferation in specialist roles. Like Taylor *et al.*'s (1994) study, this investigation also established that practitioners felt uncomfortable in performing spiritual care. Stranahan (2001, p.100) writes, 'More than half (57%) of respondents rarely or never provided spiritual care...'

The findings of all these investigations, if taken literally, imply that, despite all the attention and presumed advancement in this area, health care professionals are still struggling to recognize and engage with the concepts. However, these findings may be explained by the fact that many of the practitioners may have been providing spiritual care but not labelling it as such. The danger with elucidating and defining spiritual care is that this area of practice is fragmented and viewed as something separate to the everyday practices that health care professionals perform (Carroll 2001).

In summary, the empirical literature corroborates and substantiates the conceptual, theoretical and anecdotal evidence surrounding spirituality. It affirms that spirituality is personal, uniquely defined by individuals, and that it is dependent upon one's own personal philosophy/worldview. The studies demonstrate that spirituality may have relevance to all people, believers and non-believers. Yet, the principle of universality is precarious in the sense that the language and discourses associated with meaning are not always recognizable. For example, many patient groups linked spirituality with religious beliefs. The studies also provide valuable insight into why a group may view spirituality in a particular manner and the forces that influence their understanding – for example, Burkhardt (1991) identified and described how women in Appalachia viewed their spirituality and the societal forces that shaped this understanding, while Cavendish *et al.* (2000) used grounded theory to clarify the opportunities in life that support or enhance spirituality in well adults living in a region within the US. More recently, Shirahama and Inoue (2001) conducted an ethnographical study to explore the concept of spirituality and its expressions among persons living in a Japanese farming community. These investigations demonstrate that perceptions and understandings of spirituality may be shaped by a variety of social, cultural or regional factors such as religious beliefs, ideologies and historical associations.

While the empirical studies provide a valuable insight into how spirituality may be perceived and defined by specific populations, there was a noticeable lack of comparative studies, comparative in this instance meaning simultaneously contrasting the perceptions of two or more groups of participants – for example, nurses, patients, chaplains, physicians; or studies that have compared the perceptions of the same professional group – for example, nurses working in a variety of specialities such as critical care, palliative care, mental health, learning disabilities. It seems that many of the studies undertaken have targeted a specific group – for example, Narayanasamy, Gates and Swinton (2002) obtained critical incidents from learning disability nurses in an attempt to understand how they meet the spiritual needs of the people for whom they care. This type of research is valuable in that it provides insights into the perceptions and practices of a specific professional group. However, the results cannot be generalized to a wider audience (Carroll 2001).

The empirical literature highlights that a large proportion of the research undertaken focused upon the role of the nurse. In addition, much of the research has been conducted by nurses. However, several studies were identified within the UK that had been conducted by chaplains (O'Driscoll 2002;

Wright 2001, 2002). Only four comparative studies were identified that sought the perceptions of more than one group.

Reed (1991) used a questionnaire to explore preferences for spirituality related to nursing interventions with terminally ill and non-terminally ill hospitalised adults, contrasting their views with those of well adults. The findings of this investigation emphasized the need for nurses to be sensitive to the spiritual needs of all patients, not just those with a religious belief. Highfield (1992) investigated the spiritual health of oncology patients by contrasting nurses' and patients' perspectives. The study revealed that gender differences may be influential in undertaking an assessment of a patient's spiritual health, because males were less inclined to talk about spiritual issues. Emblen and Halstead (1993) used a descriptive qualitative design to collect interview data to establish how patients, nurses and chaplains defined spiritual needs and interventions. The findings demonstrate a need for nurses and chaplains to work collaboratively in meeting patients' spiritual needs.

Most of the comparative studies described have been conducted in the US employed quantitative or qualitative methods, or a combination of both, with the exception of Emblen and Halstead (1993) who used grounded theory. Comparative investigations are important because they shed light on the disparities and commonalities in understanding between participant groups. In addition, they provide researchers with an opportunity to explore possible reasons, explanations and potential solutions. The literature search indicates that no additional comparative studies have been undertaken in the US. The literature search reveals also that none was identified that originated within the UK. This is interesting because Ross (1997, p.714), who identified a need for such research having undertaken a pilot study of elderly patients' perceptions of their spiritual needs and care, writes:

> A study comparing both nurses' and patients' interpretations of spiritual needs and care would help clarify what spiritual needs and spiritual care are and would highlight the type of help patients might welcome with their spiritual needs.

It appears that there is an urgent need for comparative studies to investigate the discrepancies that exist between health care professionals' and patient groups' perceptions of spirituality and spiritual care. The results of such investigations could be used to inform future policy initiatives and guidelines that surround spiritual care.

The empirical literature verifies that an exclusive language of spirituality may have been created within health care. Several authors stress the need for health care professionals to avoid using and generalizing unfamiliar terminology in their dealings with patients (Hermann 2001; McSherry and Cash 2004; Taylor, Amenta and Highfield 1995). This argument could be extended also to diverse cultural groups. A major limitation of many of the studies reviewed is the lack of cultural and religious diversity. Many of the studies comprised very small samples and, because of the homogenous nature of the subjects in terms of religious belief, professional group and area of residency, these limit the generalizability of the findings.

There is a growing expectation in the empirical literature that the composition of study samples should reflect the ethnic and religious diversity that exists within a pluralistic society. With regards to investigating the spiritual dimension, there is a growing realization by researchers that the insights previously developed may not have meaning for individuals from many of the Eastern religions' traditions who, it seems, have been underrepresented in earlier research. My interpretation of this situation is that there has not been a conscious attempt to exclude such groups. On the contrary, one plausible explanation may be that the samples used have reflected the majority population working or residing in those areas at the time of conducting the investigation.

Besides, there may well have been difficulties in identifying and recruiting individuals from diverse ethnic groups due to language barriers. Other sociological factors may have been operational also – for example, perceptions of authority, how the information will be used and confidentiality if researchers are from the same ethnic group. Having stated this, there is now a pressing need to ensure that future investigations into spirituality and spiritual care do reflect the ethnic and religious diversity that exists within those regions. By including the perceptions of the minority ethnic, religious groups, a richer insight into the concept of spirituality will be gained.

Enhancement of spiritual care practices

One of the central themes identifiable within the empirical literature is linked to the enhancement of spiritual care practices. As indicated, several of the investigations have focused primarily upon the spiritual care interventions of health care professionals who were primarily nurses. The empirical literature appears judgmental of health care professionals who do not demonstrate a familiarity and fluency with the language of spirituality and the practice of spiritual care (Taylor *et al.* 1995). Enhancement of spiritual care practices can be explained by two subcategories. First, there are those investigations that make recommendations to enhance patient care by making inferences – for example, by developing the technical skills and competence of health care professionals, which will lead to improvements in spiritual care. Developing technical skills means nurturing the health care professionals' own personal awareness of spirituality in conjunction with education to develop skills to address patients' spiritual needs. Second, there are those studies that attempt to enhance spiritual care practices by offering insight into the experiential world of patients.

Several of the studies reviewed that explored health care professionals' perceptions of spirituality and spiritual care assume that deficits in relation to the provision of spiritual care may be remedied through education (Harrington 1995; Kuuppelomaki 2001; Taylor *et al.* 1994, 1995). It is assumed education will remove the discomfort and unease that some health care professionals feel when addressing spiritual needs. However, what is not explored in the educational debates is whether it is ethical to change health care professionals' perceptions of spirituality. Neither is there any real exploration of the economic or emotional cost of providing spiritual care (Walter 2002). Furthermore, an assumption seems to be made that all health care professionals want to attend, and should be attending to the spiritual needs of service users.

The empirical literature revealed a growing number of investigations that examined the spiritual well-being of specific patient or client groups. These studies focus upon individuals living with acute or chronic illness or diseased systems, such as endocrine, neurological and cardiac systems. This form of specialization is in keeping with the medical and reductionist models that prevail within health care. Clark and Heidenreich (1995) interviewed 63 patients in a critical care unit identifying nursing intervention that may enhance patients' spiritual well-being. Walton (1997) explored the relationship of spirituality in patients recovering from acute myocardial infarction and patients undergoing heart transplantation (Walton and St Clair 2000). Daalemann, Cobb and Frey (2001) used focus group interviews to elicit understandings of spirituality among female patients with type 2 diabetes and how they viewed its impact upon their health and well-being, while Arnold *et al.* (2002) used focus groups to establish patients' attitudes concerning the inclusion of spirituality into addiction treatment. More recently, Baldacchino (2002) (using combined methods) conducted a longitudinal study into the spiritual coping strategies of Maltese patients who had suffered their first acute myocardial infarction. She concludes that maintaining an individual's spiritual well-being may be a precursor to the relief of anxiety and depression. All these studies demonstrate that spirituality can be a powerful force that enables the patient to endure illness and hospitalization. In addition, these studies may highlight aspects of spiritual care that are unique to these individual groups. However, the fundamental message communicated within these investigations is the central role that health care professionals play in maintaining patients' spiritual well-being.

Activity 7.5

Do you think spirituality helps patients cope with their illness or condition? Can you think of any cases from your own practice that might confirm the research presented in this section?

A major limitation of the quantitative studies reviewed is that, while they offered valuable insight into a broad range of issues pertaining to spirituality and spiritual care, this insight was often superficial in that they were unable to convey the full extent of a participant's beliefs or feelings. The quantitative studies were not capable of exploring the complexity of the area or portray, convey the meaning, feeling and emotion that an individual or group had regarding the issue(s) under investigation. It would appear that, because of the sensitive and personal nature of spirituality, qualitative research is more suitable for exploring this dimension.

In summary, this section has highlighted limitations and omissions within existing empirical studies:

1. Investigations have been initiated principally by nurse researchers and directed mainly upon nurses' perceptions of spirituality and spiritual care practices.
2. Very few comparative studies were located that contrasted simultaneously the views of two or more groups.
3. The study samples have been homogenous reflecting the views of specific cultural, professional and client groups.
4. The quantitative studies were not really capable of exploring the complexity of spirituality.

This section outlined two central themes identifiable within the empirical literature associated with perceptions of spirituality and spiritual care. The review demonstrates that both quantitative and qualitative methods have made a significant contribution in elucidating the concept of spirituality. The section describes how quantitative studies have been significant in terms of developing insight into perceptions of spirituality and spiritual care. A limitation with some of the quantitative investigations is that they have been unable to offer a deep insight into the personal and socially constructed world of individual experience. In addition, the review suggests that few qualitative studies have been undertaken comparing and contrasting simultaneously the views of diverse groups.

Activity 7.6

What do you feel about the results of these research findings? Do you think that they have any implications for your practice?

Nurses' perceptions survey

McSherry (1998) presents the findings of a large descriptive survey of nurses of all grades working full and part time on wards in a large National Health Service Trust. This work builds upon the work of the aforementioned researchers, generating a deeper insight into how nurses perceive spirituality. A questionnaire, with covering letter, was distributed to 1029 nurses. A response rate of 55.3 per cent was obtained; the total number of questionnaires returned was 559. The questionnaire was designed to gain data that would address the research aims (Box 7.2).

The research identified that nurses perceive spirituality as a universal concept that is relevant to all individuals. Nurses are prepared to participate in the provision of spiritual care, emphasizing the need for a team approach. The nurses surveyed felt that matters concerning the spiritual dimension need to be placed firmly within existing nursing curricula. The abstract, reproduced in Box 7.3, offers a fuller insight into this research. (A copy of the questionnaire used in this study can be found in the Appendix.)

Meaning of spirituality and spiritual care

This section provides a brief summary of McSherry's (2004, pp.21–24) research investigating health care professionals', patients' and the public's perceptions of spirituality.

Box 7.2 Research aims

Explore nurses' attitudes to and perceptions of spirituality

Identify whether patients' spiritual needs are being recognized by nurses

Establish whether qualified nurses feel that they are able to meet their patients' spiritual needs

Establish whether qualified nurses feel that they receive sufficient education and training to enable them to meet patients' spiritual needs effectively

Briefly explore the possible associations that may exist between religion and nurses' understanding of spirituality and the provision of spiritual care

Box 7.3 Abstract from the nurses' perception survey

This descriptive research investigated Nurses' Perceptions of Spirituality and Spiritual Care, an area of nursing which is very personal, sensitive and shrouded in misconception and ambiguity. The study was designed to address some of these misconceptions by exploring what nurses perceive spirituality to be and how they provide spiritual care. The research was concerned with the identification of patients with spiritual needs, educational issues pertaining to spirituality, and religious practices.

The study was quantitative in design, taking the form of a descriptive survey. The Spirituality and Spiritual Care Rating Scale (SSCRS) was specifically designed for this research and was distributed to 1029 qualified and unqualified nurses working on wards in a large National Health Service Trust in East Yorkshire, England. Of the questionnaires distributed, 559 were returned giving a response rate of 55.3 per cent. The SSCRS obtained an alpha coefficient of 0.6443 for the 17–item scale and when items with low inter-item correlations were removed an alpha coefficient of 0.77 was obtained indicating an acceptable level of reliability for a newly developed instrument. The questionnaires were analysed using SPSS (Statistical Package for the Social Sciences).

Findings indicated that both qualified (392) 71.4 per cent and unqualified nurses (68) 12.3 per cent are identifying patients with spiritual needs. Of the qualified nurses who responded (219), 39.9 per cent felt that they were able to meet their patients' spiritual needs. The survey found that patients themselves would indicate to nurses the presence of a spiritual need, (372) 67.8 per cent of the nurses surveyed. These findings demonstrate that nurses are prepared to be involved in the provision of spiritual care. The results raise questions about the quality and type of spiritual care being provided since (290) 52.8 per cent of the qualified nurses stated that they had not received any instruction into the spiritual dimension. The study suggests that nurses have a willingness and desire to know more about the concept. This is evident by the large number of qualified nurses (394) 71.8 per cent who felt that they did not receive sufficient training into this aspect of care. Of the nurses surveyed (421), 76.7 per cent felt that a team approach (involving the patient, nurses, chaplains, family, friends) was needed in the provision of spiritual care indicating that nurses felt that no single profession was solely responsible. Religious beliefs and religious practices did not appear to significantly influence the provision of spiritual care. Of the nurses surveyed (409), 74.5 per cent stated that they had a religion but only (160) 29.1 per cent stated that they were practising their religion.

For the purpose of this study an Exploratory Factor Analysis was used employing Varimax rotation in an attempt to identify any underlying associations between variables in the SSCRS. This analysis suggested a 15-item instrument with four factor-based subscales: Existential Search Rudiments of Spiritual Care Universality Individuality. These factors were described and underlying associations explained in relation to existing literature. The identification of these factors suggests that the nurses surveyed had a broad universal understanding of spirituality which was relevant to all individuals irrespective of religious affiliation. The findings also indicate that nurses are aware that the provision of spiritual care is inherently different to the provision of general care.

The findings of this research validate previous British studies addressing this aspect of care (Harrison and Burnard 1993; Narayanasamy 1993; Simsen 1985; Waugh 1992). This process of validation suggests that these results may well reflect the larger population of nurses. However, caution needs to be exercised in that the SSCRS is a newly developed instrument which will need to be refined and validated by subsequent research.

Adapted from McSherry (1997), pp.2–3

In order to gain access to perceptions of spirituality held by health care professionals, patients and the general public, and to information about the extent to which they expect to either provide or receive spiritual care, I used a qualitative research method. A grounded theory investigation was undertaken, using semi-structured interviews. These were conducted with a sample of health care professionals, patients and members of the public who were neither patients nor health care professionals but came from particular faith communities. The investigation took place between September 1998 and August 2003. This time frame included theoretical and methodological preparation, prior to data collection, as well as data collection and analysis.

The investigation was undertaken in three areas:

- Area I (a hospice)
- Area II (a large Acute National Health Service Trust)
- Area III (a large Acute National Health Service Trust).

Areas I and III were situated in the same city in the North of England. Area II was in another city in the same geographical region. Using two different regions allowed me to capture the ethnic and religious diversity that existed. Area II was specifically selected because from the last national census (Office for National Statistics 2001) the region contained a greater diversity of ethnic groups than the region in which Areas I and III were situated.

ETHICAL APPROVAL

Before data collection commenced, ethical approval was obtained from the relevant Local Research Ethics Committee.

DATA COLLECTION

Initial approval to start data collection was made in the first area in July 2000, followed by data collection, analysis and the writing of the merging theory. In line with the grounded theory approach adopted, all these activities were undertaken in a cyclical manner throughout the duration of the investigation.

The interviews (semi-structured) were conducted in three phases:

Phase 1 explored participants' perceptions and understandings of the term 'spirituality'. It was conducted principally with patients and nurses from the hospice, who identified their willingness to participate by responding positively to a question on the questionnaire about their views of spirituality. This phase suggested that there might be major differences in the way that, as groups of individuals, patients and nurses understood the word 'spirituality'. Several patients had no real understanding about what the word meant –

indeed, some had never even heard of the word; more surprisingly, some of the representatives from a number of the major religions also seemed to have difficulty understanding it. This finding resulted in the need to conduct Phase 2.

Phase 2 was carried out with nurses and patients in the two Acute Trusts. In this phase, a number of questions were asked in order to determine whether patients and nurses would recognize the constituents of spirituality as expressed in the health care literature. For example, participants were asked to comment upon what provided their life with meaning, purpose and fulfilment. They were also asked whether they considered that these aspects of their lives were part of spirituality. This phase helped to develop further insights into how participants viewed spirituality. In addition, it revealed that spiritual care was provided by a number of health care professions; interestingly, it also suggested that nurses feel that no single professional group has a monopoly regarding this area of practice. These findings led to the development of Phase 3.

In Phase 3, the findings from Phases 1 and 2 were explored with a number of health care professionals, including a social worker, two physiotherapists and seven chaplains, who were recruited from Area I and Area III. These groups were perceived by participants in the previous phases as being responsible for the provision of spiritual care.

In this phase, several aspects of the theory that had begun to be developed in the previous phases were tested out and substantiated. These were that the word 'spirituality' was not recognized by all participants; that not all the constituents of spirituality were recognized as such by all participants; and that not all patients or members of the public had an expectation that spiritual care would be provided as part of health care.

During this phase it was noticed that not all the major world religions had been represented. As a result, a member of the Jewish community was recruited (from the Orthodox tradition).

The three phases of the investigation led to the creation of the theory titled 'assumption versus expectation' and the creation of a model for advancing understanding of spirituality and spiritual care within health care.

Summary of the main research findings and limitations

The studies reviewed investigating health care professionals' perceptions of spirituality and spiritual care demonstrate that there is still a fundamental need to establish how individuals *interpret* and *define* spirituality and spiritual care.

Box 7.4 The meaning of spirituality and spiritual care: an investigation of health care professionals', patients' and public's perceptions

This Grounded Theory investigation explored health care professionals' (Health care professionals), patients' and public's perceptions of spirituality and spiritual care. The investigation had three objectives: to examine the assumption that spirituality is a universally recognized and understood concept within nursing and health care; to develop insight into Health care professionals, patients' and public's understanding of spirituality and spiritual care; through constant comparative analysis in conjunction with a selected review of the literature produce a model of spirituality for health care.

Fifty three participants (24 men and 29 women) were recruited from a hospice and two large Acute National Health Service Trusts in Yorkshire, England. The sample included nursing (n = 24), chaplaincy (n = 7), social work (n = 1), occupational therapy (n = 1), physiotherapy (n = 2), patients (n = 14), public (n = 4). The investigation was conducted in three phases. In Phase I the assumption that spirituality is a universally recognized and understood concept was explored resulting in the formation of five subcategories. During Phase II participants' understanding of the components considered by Health care professionals to be important aspects of spirituality such as relationships, forgiveness, and creativity were investigated. This led to the formation of two further categories: spiritual narratives and subconscious awareness of spirituality. Phase III drew on the findings of phase I and II resulting in the creation of the 'Principle Components Model'. It is envisaged that this model will assist the development of spirituality and spiritual care within health care, education and practice. The core category titled 'assumption versus expectation' was created because it had significance for all categories and was identifiable within all phases.

The findings validate existing conceptual and theoretical constructs of spirituality promulgated within health care. This endorses the unease being expressed in some quarters that health care has created its own professional discourse in terms of language and terminology. The idea of a professional discourse was substantiated on the basis that the majority of the patient and public participants did not identify with the concept of spirituality nor did they have any real expectations in terms of receiving spiritual care. The findings reinforce a need for health care professionals to evaluate and revise the professional discourse it has seemingly created.

Source: McSherry (2004), pp.7–8

The studies undertaken have developed some insight and understanding of spiritual needs and spiritual care, yet there is an apparent lack of research focusing primarily upon how the concept of spirituality is perceived within diverse faith and world communities. The studies have focused upon health care professionals' ability to define and meet spiritual needs, and upon the provision of spiritual care. Many of the studies have targeted specific populations of, say, nurses working in oncology and surgical units, or chaplains. There is a need to investigate all health care professionals' perceptions working within *all specialties*, in order to gain a wider understanding. By extending the boundaries of investigation, a more comprehensive picture of how nurses perceive the spiritual dimension will be obtained.

Spirituality and health care professionals' education

This section introduces the educational issues surrounding the concept of spirituality, exploring how and if it should be taught within health care professionals' programmes of education. Several of the research studies mentioned earlier in this chapter have indicated a fundamental need for spirituality to be formally integrated within programmes of education. This need has been recognized and addressed within the US, and to a lesser degree within the UK, and it seems in many countries that the process of integration has been extremely slow despite researchers and educators drawing attention to this omission within existing curricula.

During the course of your own professional education you may or may not have received any formal education into the spiritual dimension. McSherry's (1997, 2004) research indicated that some nurses and, more latterly, health care professionals received some educational instruction while others received limited instruction surrounding religious practices or a talk from the hospital chaplain. At present within the UK, there is no uniform policy that explicitly states spirituality should be taught to all health care professionals, nor are there any real guidelines on what or how it should be taught. It would appear that the teaching of spirituality is left very much to the devices of individual institutions or academics who have an interest in the subject. Ironically, the competency statements that nurses, and I am sure other health care professionals, should achieve for registration imply that a student nurse should be able to assess, plan, implement and evaluate spiritual care (NMC 2002). The dilemma is how students, or indeed any health care professional, are to provide spiritual care if they do not receive some form of educational preparation that may generate insight and self-awareness.

Activity 7.7

Spend several minutes reflecting upon your own programme of education. This could be either pre-qualifying or education undertaken as part of your continuing professional development. Write down any education that you received that addressed the subject of spirituality or spiritual care.

Emerging and continuing debates

Bradshaw (1997) suggests a need for caution in relation to the teaching of spirituality in that the concept is not something that can be taught by theoretical or experiential analysis but rather that spiritual awareness comes about through clinical experience and exposure. The growing debate is whether spirituality should be 'taught' or is it something that is 'caught' in practice? Bradshaw warns that the danger of teaching about spirituality is that it becomes another component that is added into nursing curricula, thus fragmenting the individual and defeating the notion of holistic care.

If spirituality is not taught by traditional methods and it is left to be 'caught' by nurses or indeed health care professionals in practice, then there is the danger that spiritual awareness may not be generated or developed. The process of socialization and skill acquisition that is dependent upon supervision and exposure in practice may result in patients' or service users' spiritual needs not being addressed by health care professionals in practice. The problem with acquiring skills through exposure and experience may mean that neophyte nurses model and shape their practice by observing and imitating the behaviours and practices displayed by their superiors. If such role models do not address the spiritual dimension of their patients or service users, then this could result in the cycle being perpetuated and individuals' spiritual needs will constantly be neglected. However, if neophyte health care professionals have some insight into the spiritual dimension, they will be able to recognize a spiritual need when it arises, and they will possibly address the perceived need despite the inherent pressures of going against the grain.

To illustrate this point, think of an occasion(s) when as a student or a neophyte practitioner in clinical practice you were given instruction into the spiritual dimension, or can you recall when you last observed your mentor or preceptor provide an aspect of spiritual care? Bradshaw's concerns are justified in that she does not want to see spirituality as something of an amendment or an addition to the individual, but rather as a set of characteristics that is acquired through exposure in practice, as occurred in the 'old' apprenticeship style of training.

Activity 7.8

Spend several minutes reflecting upon the emerging debates, writing down what you feel are the pros and cons of both sides. Can you think of any solutions that may be a way forward?

Formal integration

During the late 1980s and early 1990s, nurse educators in the UK, and, it must be stressed, other professional groups such as those within medicine and social work in the US, have campaigned relentlessly for the formal integration of the subject of spirituality within programmes of education (Burnard 1990; Harrison and Burnard 1993; McSherry and Draper 1997; Narayanasamy 1993; Ross 1996). Ross (1996, p.43) writes:

> Guidelines for nurse education stress the need to teach spiritual care to nurses but it is not clear how the subject should be taught or how effective any teaching is in helping nurses to give spiritual care.

This quotation supports previous claims for formal integration while highlighting a need for guidelines on how this might be achieved from nursing and health care professional regulatory bodies.

There is a need for health care educators (that is those who are responsible for educating health care professionals) to take a step back and review the situation in the light of all the evidence and debates that are developing. The process of integration may not be that simple because there are several barriers that must be considered in any curriculum innovation (McSherry and Draper 1997). One major barrier is that curriculum review is often slow and it is hard to balance the content of the curriculum. If something is to be added, then often it means something else has to be shortened or removed.

However, over two decades ago, Carson and Gerardi (1985) introduced a course called 'Spirituality in Nursing Practice' within a nursing faculty in a secular university in the US with relatively good success and positive evaluations from students. Similarly within the UK, individuals with a keen interest have undertaken similar innovations designing modules, workshops, study days and conferences in order to generate awareness of the importance of spirituality within health care. These innovations and labours would be strengthened if there were consistency and unity – i.e. some form of central control indicating content, methods and importantly assessment of what should and should not be taught, instead of leaving it to an ad hoc basis. Yet some insight and education is probably better than none at all.

Teaching methods

Bradshaw (1996) is right in that spirituality as a subject is deeply personal, sensitive and highly subjective. Because of this, most of the issues associated with the subject do not lend themselves to many of the formal methods of classroom teaching.

Several nurse educators have offered suggestions as to the methods that may be suitable for the exploration of the spiritual dimension by nurses (Bush 1999; Burnard 1988; Harrison and Burnard 1993). It would appear that an important factor is the fostering of a teaching environment that is safe and confidential where students or delegates can explore spiritual issues, feeling supported and secure. One of the major concerns in many of the health care professions is the large increase in student numbers associated with intakes of between 30 and 100 students. Some subjects by their very nature can be addressed in the confines of a lecture and delivered to large audiences. However, matters surrounding spirituality are best delivered in groups of between 6 and 15. Any larger size makes facilitation difficult for the teacher.

Throughout this book, many situations have been presented that have asked for reflection – generating insight into one's own feelings and attitudes towards a specific matter. These workshop activities appear to generate discussion and debate when addressing matters concerning spirituality within the classroom. Therefore group work, reflection and exercises that generate self-awareness are more suitable for exploring the personal, sensitive and subjective aspects of spirituality. The didactic nature of formal lectures makes them unsuitable for addressing the spiritual dimension.

Activity 7.9

Spend several minutes reflecting upon your own educational experiences – how do you feel spirituality should be taught to your discipline or profession? Which type of teaching methods do you think might assist you in acquiring these skills and knowledge?

Duration

The length of time spent delivering and addressing matters concerning spirituality in any module, programme or curriculum requires careful deliberation. It is very unrealistic to think that everything there is to know about spirituality and the provision of spiritual care can be presented in sufficient depth in a 2- or 3-hour lecture. Therefore, when considering the formal integration of spirituality into existing health care curricula, this important issue must be raised (Box 7.5 presents the outline of a 2-day course addressing spirituality and spiritual care). Spirituality may be addressed within the confines of a single module or be revisited throughout the 3–5 year training programme as a major theme that is revisited within the boundaries of different modules such as theory, communication skills, legal and ethical, multicultural issues or death and dying. Adopting this approach would help alleviate some of the concerns that spirituality is seen as an afterthought.

Facilitator

The question of who should teach matters associated with spirituality is an important point that requires considerable thought and attention. In the past, spirituality was usually addressed by an hour or two in the company of the hospital chaplain. However, in a changing educational climate and a society that is now culturally and religiously diverse and, it could be argued, still sceptical of formal religious practice, how feasible is it to rely solely upon the hospital chaplain? Yet many hospital chaplains are ecumenical or 'generic' in that they provide pastoral and spiritual support to individuals from a range of religious affiliations and those with none. Perhaps a way forward is to introduce a team approach to the teaching of the spiritual dimension. It must be

Box 7.5 Outline of a 2-day course, 'Introduction to the spiritual dimensions of health care practice'

Day 1

09.30–11.00	Introduction Outline of the two days Introductory task (Task A)
11.00–11.20	Break (refreshments available)
11.20–12.30	Group work – using case studies (Task B)
12.30–13.00	Recap of morning session
13.00–14.00	Lunch
14.00–15.00	Spirituality: an exploration of the concept
15.00–15.20	Break (refreshments available)
15.20–16.20	Skills required by health care professionals to address spiritual needs (a counselling approach)
16.20–16.30	Evaluation of Day 1

Day 2

09.30–11.00	Spirituality and a systematic approach (practical session using case studies)
11.00–11.20	Break (refreshments available)
11.20–12.40	Feedback from group exercise: look at barriers that prevent nurses from implementing spiritual care
12.40–13.00	Recap of morning session
13.00–14.00	Lunch
14.00–15.00	An exploration of some of the institutional religions
15.00–15.20	Break (refreshments available)
15.20–16.20	Support networks (discussion)
16.20–16.30	Evaluation of Day 2

emphasized that the teaching of matters surrounding spirituality is very demanding and tiring in that it places a great demand on the emotional, psychological and spiritual reserve of the teacher (McSherry 2000). The individuals who teach the subject must have awareness and a degree of acceptance with their own spirituality in order to offer support to others. The notion of team teaching helps to reduce the emotional and spiritual demands placed upon one individual while drawing upon the expertise of others.

Competency

The idea of health care professionals being competent with spiritual care is very much in vogue. Within the health care literature, and indeed as indicated at the outset of this book, some professional regulatory bodies such as the Nursing and Midwifery Council and the Quality Assurance Agency are setting and monitoring the achievement of spiritual care competencies. The result of such developments is that there now seem to be constant calls for all health care professionals to be educated in spiritual matters. These appeals suggest that education and knowledge may better equip health care professionals to be more competent in dealing with spiritual matters. Some pioneering work undertaken by van Leeuwen and Cusveller (2004) presents a number of competencies for spiritual care that fall into three broad domains: awareness and use of self; spiritual dimensions of nursing; and assurance of quality and expertise. These three broad domains and their associated competencies originate out of a review of the nursing literature. There are limitations with this proposed competency framework, which the authors duly acknowledge; nevertheless, it is a valuable attempt to identify the knowledge and skills that nurses and indeed all health care professionals require to deal with patients' or service users' spiritual needs.

Similarly, Kerry (2001) wrote a useful book chapter titled 'Towards competence: a narrative and framework for spiritual care givers' outlining how competency frameworks may make a significant contribution in meeting clinical governance initiatives, adding that they may even improve the performance of chaplains assisting with the integration of spiritual care within contemporary health care. Both these pieces of work highlight how competency frameworks may help health care professionals to develop their knowledge and expertise in dealing with spiritual issues. However, the notion of competency in relation to spiritual care is still very much in its infancy and frameworks like those mentioned need to be tested to establish whether they actually lead to health care professionals being better equipped to deal with patients' spiritual concerns.

Conclusion

This chapter has introduced you to aspects of the spiritual dimension that have been investigated by health care professionals. The results generated indicate that spirituality is recognized and fundamental to individuals' health and sense of well-being. The studies provide a deeper insight into how health care professionals and patients perceive the concepts of spirituality and spiritual care. As more research is undertaken, evidence is emerging that will inform and develop health care practice, leading to improvements in the quality of spiritual care provided. As more research is undertaken into the spiritual dimension and 'old' research disseminated and evaluated, this should directly influence the way that spirituality is addressed within programmes of education. The fact that individuals are generating debate and discussion that is international is positive. The wheels of change are slow but, through perseverance and empirical research, the spiritual dimension will continue to gain prominence and remain as a focus of enquiry within health care.

Box 7.6 Final thought

Spend some time reflecting upon the main findings of the studies that have been presented in this chapter and write down what implications they have for you in the way that spiritual care is provided by you or your colleagues.

References

Arnold, R.M., Avants, S.K., Margolin, A. and Marcotte, D. (2002) 'Patients' attitudes concerning the inclusion of spirituality into addiction treatment.' *Journal of Substance Abuse Treatment 23*, 319–326.

Baldacchino, D. (2002) 'Spiritual coping of Maltese patients with first acute myocardial infarction: a longitudinal study.' Unpublished PhD thesis, Hull: University of Hull.

Baldacchino, D.R. and Buhagiar, A. (2003) 'Psychometric evaluation of the Spiritual Coping Strategies Scale in English, Maltese, back-translation and bilingual versions.' *Journal of Advanced Nursing 42*, 6, 558–570.

Bradshaw, A. (1996) 'The legacy of Nightingale.' *Nursing Times 92*, 6, 42–43.

Bradshaw, A. (1997) 'Teaching spiritual care to nurses: an alternative approach.' *International Journal of Palliative Nursing 3,* 1, 51–57.

Burkhardt, M.A. (1991) 'Exploring understandings of spirituality among women in Appalachia.' Doctoral dissertation, Florida: University of Miami.

Burkhardt, M.A. (1994) 'Becoming and connecting: elements of spirituality for women.' *Holistic Nursing Practice 8,* 4, 12–21.

Burnard, P. (1988) *Searching for meaning.' Nursing Times 84,* 37, 34–36.

Burnard, P. (1990) 'Learning to care for the spirit.' *Nursing Standard 4,* 18, 38–39.

Bush, T. (1999) 'Journalling and the teaching of spirituality.' *Nurse Education Today 19,* 20–28.

Carroll, B. (2001) 'A phenomenological exploration of the nature of spirituality and spiritual care.' *Morality 6,* 1, 81–98.

Carson, V. and Gerardi, R. (1985) 'Spirituality for credit: finding a place in the secular curriculum.' *Journal of Christian Nursing 2,* 3, 28–30.

Cavendish, R., Luise, B.K., Horne, K., Bauer, M., Medefindt, G.M.A., Calvino, C. and Kutza, T. (2000) 'Opportunities for enhanced spirituality relevant to well adults.' *Nursing Diagnosis 11,* 4, 151–163.

Chiu, L. (2001) 'Spiritual resources of Chinese immigrants with breast cancer in the USA.' *International Journal of Nursing Studies 38,* 175–184.

Clark, C. and Heidenreich, T. (1995) 'Spiritual care for the critically ill American.' *Journal of Critical Care 4,* 1, 77–81.

Conco, D. (1995) 'Christian patients' views of spiritual care.' *Western Journal of Nursing Research 17,* 3, 266–276.

Conrad, N.L. (1985) 'Spiritual support for the dying.' *Nursing Clinics of North America 20,* 2, 415–426.

Daalemann, T.P., Cobb, A.K. and Frey, B.B. (2001) 'Spirituality and well-being: an exploratory study of the patient perspective.' *Social Science and Medicine 53,* 1503–1511.

Dunn, P.M. (1993) 'An investigation into the concept of spiritual needs of hospitalised patients, from a nursing perspective.' Unpublished dissertation, Institute of Nursing Studies, Hull: University of Hull.

Emblen, J.D. and Halstead, L. (1993) Spiritual needs and interventions: comparing the views of patients, nurses and chaplains.' *Clinical Nurse Specialist 7,* 4, 175–182.

Hall, T.W. and Edwards, K.J. (2002) 'The spiritual assessment inventory: a theistic model and measure for assessing spiritual development.' *Journal of Scientific Study of Religion 41,* 2, 341–357.

Harrington, A. (1995) 'Spiritual care: what does it mean to RNs?' *Australian Journal of Advanced Nursing 12,* 4, 5–14.

Harrison, J. and Burnard, P. (1993) *Spirituality and Nursing Practice.* Aldershot: Avebury.

Hermann, C.P. (2001) 'Spiritual needs of dying patients: a qualitative study.' *Oncology Nursing Forum 28,* 1, 67–72.

Highfield, M.F. (1992) 'Spiritual health of oncology patients: nurse and patient perspectives.' *Cancer Nursing 15*, 1, 1–8.

Kearney, S. (1994) 'Spirituality as a coping mechanism in multiple sclerosis: the patient's perspective.' Unpublished dissertation, Hull: Institute of Nursing Studies, University of Hull.

Kerry, M. (2001) 'Towards competence: a narrative and framework for spiritual care givers.' In H. Orchard (ed.) (2001) *Spirituality in Health Care Contexts*, 118–132. London: Jessica Kingsley Publishers.

Kuuppelomaki, M. (2001) 'Spiritual support for terminally ill patients: nursing staff assessments.' *Journal of Clinical Nursing 10*, 660–670.

McSherry, W. (1997) 'A descriptive survey of nurses' perceptions of spirituality and spiritual care.' Unpublished MPhil thesis, Hull: University of Hull.

McSherry, W. (1998) 'Nurses' perceptions of spirituality and spiritual care.' *Nursing Standard 13*, 4, 36–40.

McSherry, W. (2000) 'Educational issues surrounding the teaching of spirituality.' *Nursing Standard 14*, 42, 40–43.

McSherry, W. (2004) 'The meaning of spirituality and spiritual care: an investigation of health care professionals', patients' and public's perceptions.' Unpublished PhD thesis, Leeds: Leeds Metropolitan University.

McSherry, W. and Cash, K. (2004) 'The language of spirituality: an emerging taxonomy.' *International Journal of Nursing Studies 41*, 151–161.

McSherry, W. and Draper, P. (1997) 'The spiritual dimension: why the absence within nursing curricula?' *Nurse Education Today 17*, 413–417.

McSherry, W., Draper, P. and Kendrick, D. (2002) 'The construct validity of a rating scale designed to assess spirituality and spiritual care International.' *Journal of Nursing Studies 39*, 7, 723–734.

Narayanasamy, A. (1993) 'Nurses' awareness and educational preparation in meeting their patients' spiritual needs.' *Nurse Education Today 13*, 3, 196–201.

Narayanasamy, A. (2002) 'Spiritual coping mechanisms in chronically ill patients.' *British Journal of Nursing 11*, 21, 1461–1470.

Narayanasamy, A. and Owens, J. (2001) 'A critical incident study of nurses' responses to the spiritual needs of their patients.' *Journal of Advanced Nursing 33*, 4, 446–455.

Narayanasamy, A., Gates, B. and Swinton, J. (2002) 'Spirituality and learning disabilities: a qualitative study British.' *Journal of Nursing 11*, 14, 948–957.

Nursing and Midwifery Council (NMC) (2002) 'Requirements for pre-registration nursing programmes.' London: NMC.

O'Driscoll, P.J. (2002) 'A study of the perceptions and understanding of spirituality and spiritual care of the nurses of the Basildon and Thurrock General Hospitals Trust.' Unpublished MA dissertation, Leeds: The University of Leeds.

Office for National Statistics (2002) Census 2001. London: HMSO. Available at: www.statistics.gov.uk/census/2001.

Paloutzian, R.F. and Ellison, C.W. (1979) 'Developing a measure of spiritual well-being.' In R.F. Paloutzian (chair) *Spiritual Well-being, Loneliness and Perceived Quality of life.* Symposium presented at the annual meeting of the American Psychological Association, New York.

Reed, P.R. (1991) 'Preferences for spirituality related nursing interventions among terminally ill and non-terminally ill hospitalised adults and well adults.' *Applied Nursing Research 4,* 3, 122–128.

Ross, L.A. (1996) 'Teaching spiritual care to nurses.' *Nurse Education Today 16,* 38–43.

Ross, L.A. (1997) 'Elderly patients' perceptions of their spiritual needs and care: a pilot study.' *Journal of Advanced Nursing 26,* 710–715.

Shirahama, K. and Inoue E.M. (2001) 'Spirituality in nursing from a Japanese perspective.' *Holistic Nursing Practice 15,* 3, 63–72.

Simsen, B. (1985) 'Spiritual needs and resources in illness and hospitalisation.' Unpublished MSc thesis, Manchester: University of Manchester.

Stranahan, S. (2001) 'Spiritual perceptions, attitudes about spiritual care, and spiritual care practices among nurse practitioners.' *Western Journal of Nursing Research 23,* 1, 90–104.

Strang, S. and Strang, P. (2001) 'Spiritual thoughts, coping and "sense of coherence" in brain tumour patients and their spouses.' *Palliative Medicine 15,* 127–134.

Taylor, E.J. (2003) 'Nurses caring for the spirit: patients with cancer and family caregiver expectations.' *Oncology Nursing Forum 30,* 4, 585–590.

Taylor, E.J., Amenta, M. and Highfield, M. (1995) 'Spiritual care practices of oncology nurses.' *Oncology Nurses Forum 22,* 1, 31–39.

Taylor, E.J., Highfield, M. and Amenta, M. (1994) 'Attitudes and beliefs regarding spiritual care: a survey of cancer nurses.' *Cancer Nursing 17,* 6, 479–487.

Taylor, E.J. and Mariner, I. (2005) 'Spiritual care nursing: what cancer patients and family caregivers want.' *Journal of Advanced Nursing 49,* 3, 260–267.

Thomas, J. and Retsas, A. (1999) 'Transacting self-preservation: a grounded theory of the spiritual dimension of people with terminal cancer.' *International Journal of Nursing Studies 36,* 3, 191–201.

Tuck, I., McCain, N.L. and Elswick, R.K. (2001) 'Spirituality and psychosocial factors in persons living with HIV.' *Journal of Advanced Nursing 33,* 6, 776–783.

van Leeuwen, R. and Cusveller, B. (2004) 'Nursing competencies for spiritual care.' *Journal of Advanced Nursing 48,* 3, 234–246.

Walter, T. (2002) 'Spirituality in palliative care: opportunity or burden?' *Palliative Medicine 16,* 133–139.

Walton, J. (1997) 'Spirituality of patients recovering from an acute myocardial infarction: a grounded theory study.' Unpublished doctoral dissertation, Kansas City: University of Missouri.

Walton, J. (1999) 'Spirituality of patients recovering from an acute myocardial infarction: a grounded theory study.' *Journal of Holistic Nursing 17,* 1, 34–53.

Walton, J. and St Clair, K. (2000) '"A beacon of light" spirituality in the heart transplant patient.' *Critical Care Nursing Clinics of North America 12*, 1, 87–101.

Waugh, L.A. (1992) 'Spiritual aspects of nursing: a descriptive study of nurses' perceptions.' Unpublished PhD thesis, Edinburgh: Queen Margaret College.

Wright, M.C. (2001) 'Chaplaincy in hospice and hospital: findings from a survey in England and Wales.' *Palliative Medicine 15*, 229–242.

Wright, M.C. (2002) 'The essence of spiritual care: a phenomenological enquiry.' *Palliative Medicine 16*, 125–132.

Further reading

Research texts

Any of these texts will provide the reader with a detailed insight into the different approaches to research and the stages involved in the research process. However, you may want to identify if any research tests have been written specifically for your own health care profession.

Burns, N. and Grove, S.K. (1997) *The Practice of Nursing Research Conduct, Critique and Utilization*, 3rd edn. Philadelphia: WB Saunders.

Malterud, K. (2001) 'Qualitative research: standards, challenges, and guidelines.' *The Lancet 358*, August 11, 483–488.

Polit, D.F. and Hungler, B.P. (1999) *Nursing Research Principles and Methods*, 6th edn. Philadelphia: Lippincott.

Research studies addressing perceptions of spirituality

Readers are encouraged to look at other international studies referenced throughout the chapter for a global appreciation of how spirituality and spiritual care are being investigated.

Spirituality and education

The following texts will bring the reader up to date with the growing debate addressing spirituality within health care education. The reader is also encouraged to look at other international studies that have been referenced throughout the chapter for a more global appreciation.

Bradshaw, A. (1997) 'Teaching spiritual care to nurses: an alternative approach.' *International Journal of Palliative Nursing 3*, 1, 51–57.

Burnard, P. (1990) 'Learning to care for the spirit.' *Nursing Standard 4*, 18, 38–39.

Furman, L.D., Benson, P.W., Grimwood, C. and Canda, E. (2004) 'Religion and spirituality in social work education and direct practice at the millennium: a survey of UK social works.' *British Journal of Social Work 34*, 767–792.

Greenstreet, W. (1999) 'Teaching spirituality in nursing: a literature review.' *Nurse Education Today 19*, 649–658.

Kerry, M. (2001) 'Towards competence: a narrative and framework for spiritual care givers.' In H. Orchard (ed.) (2001) *Spirituality in Health Care Contexts*, 118–132. London: Jessica Kingsley Publishers.

McSherry, W. (2000) 'Educational issues surrounding the teaching of spirituality.' *Nursing Standard 14*, 42, 40–43.

McSherry, W. and Draper, P. (1997) 'The spiritual dimension: why the absence within nursing curricula?' *Nurse Education Today 17*, 413–417.

Narayanasamy, A. (1993) 'Nurses' awareness and educational preparation in meeting their patients' spiritual needs.' *Nurse Education Today 13*, 3, 196–201.

Narayanasamy, A. (1999) 'Learning spiritual dimensions of care from a historical perspective.' *Nurse Education Today 19*, 386–395.

Ross, L.A. (1996) 'Teaching spiritual care to nurses.' *Nurse Education Today 16*, 38–43.

van Leeuwen, R. and Cusveller, B. (2004) 'Nursing competencies for spiritual care.' *Journal of Advanced Nursing 48*, 3, 234–246.

APPENDIX

Spirituality and Spiritual Care Rating Scale

Introduction

Research into spirituality is discussed in detail in Chapter 7. The rating scale used by McSherry (1997) is described in this Appendix, and the text of the questionnaire used to provide a spirituality and spiritual care rating scale (SSCRS) is reproduced in full.

Notes on construction

As you are aware, the concept of spirituality is very broad and subjective. Therefore, if an individual respondent were simply asked to write down what he or she thought spirituality was, some might well be able to write a thesis. To prevent this and to make statistical analysis easier, the rating scale was devised and constructed covering key areas associated with spirituality and spiritual care. The material for these questions was identified in the literature. Questions were then formulated and constructed.

The 23-item scale was structured around nine fundamental areas pertaining to spirituality (Box A.1) that have been documented or identified in the literature by several authors (Carson 1989; Emblen and Halstead 1993; Frankl 1987; Harrison and Burnard 1993; Narayanasamy 1991; Shelly and Fish 1988; Waugh 1992). It was around the work of these key authors that the framework for the SSCRS was designed and structured.

The rating scale was constructed using a five-point Likert scale. A five-point scale was chosen because more complex scoring methods had been shown to possess no advantage (Oppenheim 1992, p.195). Respondents were asked to circle their preferred answer. Scoring was as described in Box A.2.

Originally a 23-item pool was formulated. In the first draft, the Ethics Committee felt that the items seemed to follow on from each other in sequence – a response-set bias. In order to address this possible response set, the 17 items used in the final rating scale were randomized using random number tables and

Box A.1 Fundamental areas pertaining to spirituality

1 Hope
2 Meaning and purpose
3 Forgiveness
4 Beliefs and values
5 Spiritual care
6 Relationships
7 Belief in a God or deity
8 Morality
9 Creativity and self-expression

Box A.2 Scoring for the scale

1 = Strongly disagree

2 = Disagree

3 = Uncertain

4 = Agree

5 = Strongly agree

individualized. This meant that each item began with 'I believe spirituality…' or 'I believe nurses can provide spiritual care by…'. In order to prevent any response-set bias, 25 per cent of the 23 items were phrased in the negative, e.g. 'I believe spirituality is not concerned with a belief and faith in a God or supreme being'. These measures taken to prevent a response-set bias appeared to be effective. When the 23 items were analysed after the pre-pilot phases, six items were found not to be contributing to the overall scores in a significant way; these were removed from the item pool. Originally the SSCRS was designed in two parts: questions a-q addressed elements of spirituality and questions r-w addressed issues pertaining to spiritual care. Eventually all the questions in the scale were randomized and integrated. Integrating questions was another measure taken to try and prevent any response-set bias. For a more in-depth exploration into the construction of the scale please consult the following paper: McSherry, W., Draper, P. and Kendrick, D. (2002) 'The construct validity of a rating scale designed to assess spirituality and spiritual care.' *International Journal of Nursing Studies 39*, 7, 723–734.

It is anticipated that the SSCRS can be used by researchers investigating the spiritual dimension.

Update

Since the scale's construction and subsequent publication, I have received 31 requests to use it primarily within research investigations. It has been used in China, Portugal, Taiwan, Turkey, the US and the UK. I am currently undertaking research using the above scale with a view to using Confirmatory Factor Analysis to refine and establish the scale as a measure in determining an individual's perceptions of spirituality and spiritual care. Interestingly, some of the results that I have received from these studies demonstrate that the scale possesses good levels of validity and reliability. A study undertaken by O'Driscoll (2002) produced similar findings to those obtained in my original survey (McSherry 1997). Details of this study are: O'Driscoll, P.J. (2002) 'A study of the perceptions and understanding of spirituality and spiritual care of the nurses of the Basildon and Thurrock General Hospitals Trust.' Unpublished MA dissertation, Leeds: The University of Leeds.

Spirituality and spiritual care rating scale (SSCRS)

For each question please circle one answer that best reflects the extent to which you agree or disagree with each statement.

a) I believe nurses can provide spiritual care by arranging a visit by the hospital chaplain or the patient's own religious leader if requested.

Strongly disagree	Disagree	Uncertain	Agree	Strongly agree
1	2	3	4	5

b) I believe nurses can provide spiritual care by showing kindness, concern and cheerfulness when giving care.

Strongly disagree	Disagree	Uncertain	Agree	Strongly agree
1	2	3	4	5

c) I believe spirituality is concerned with a need to forgive and a need to be forgiven.

Strongly disagree	Disagree	Uncertain	Agree	Strongly agree
1	2	3	4	5

d) I believe spirituality involves only going to church/place of worship.

Strongly disagree	Disagree	Uncertain	Agree	Strongly agree
1	2	3	4	5

e) I believe spirituality is not concerned with a belief and faith in a God or Supreme Being.

Strongly disagree	Disagree	Uncertain	Agree	Strongly agree
1	2	3	4	5

f) I believe spirituality is about finding meaning in the good and bad events of life.

Strongly disagree	Disagree	Uncertain	Agree	Strongly agree
1	2	3	4	5

g) I believe nurses can provide spiritual care by spending time with a patient, giving support and reassurance especially in time of need.

Strongly disagree	Disagree	Uncertain	Agree	Strongly agree
1	2	3	4	5

h) I believe nurses can provide spiritual care by enabling a patient to find meaning and purpose in his or her illness.

Strongly disagree	Disagree	Uncertain	Agree	Strongly agree
1	2	3	4	5

i) I believe spirituality is about having a sense of hope in life.

Strongly disagree	Disagree	Uncertain	Agree	Strongly agree
1	2	3	4	5

j) I believe spirituality is to do with the way one conducts one's life here and now.

Strongly disagree	Disagree	Uncertain	Agree	Strongly agree
1	2	3	4	5

k) I believe nurses can provide spiritual care by listening to and allowing patients time to discuss and explore their fears, anxieties and troubles.

Strongly disagree	Disagree	Uncertain	Agree	Strongly agree
1	2	3	4	5

l) I believe spirituality is a unifying force which enables one to be at peace with oneself and the world.

Strongly disagree	Disagree	Uncertain	Agree	Strongly agree
1	2	3	4	5

m) I believe spirituality does not include areas such as art, creativity and self-expression.

Strongly disagree	Disagree	Uncertain	Agree	Strongly agree
1	2	3	4	5

n) I believe nurses can provide spiritual care by having respect for privacy, dignity and religious and cultural beliefs of a patient.

Strongly disagree	Disagree	Uncertain	Agree	Strongly agree
1	2	3	4	5

o) I believe spirituality involves personal friendships and relationships.

Strongly disagree	Disagree	Uncertain	Agree	Strongly agree
1	2	3	4	5

p) I believe spirituality does not apply to atheists or agnostics.

Strongly disagree	Disagree	Uncertain	Agree	Strongly agree
1	2	3	4	5

q) I believe spirituality includes people's morals.

Strongly disagree	Disagree	Uncertain	Agree	Strongly agree
1	2	3	4	5

Copyright © Wilfred McSherry 2005
For permission to use the SSCRS, please contact Wilfred McSherry at:
Faculty of Health and Social Care
The University of Hull
Cottingham Road
Hull HU6 7RX, UK

References

Carson, V.B. (1989) *Spiritual Dimensions of Nursing Practice.* Philadelphia: WB Saunders.

Emblen, J.D. and L. Halstead (1993) 'Spiritual needs and interventions: comparing the views of patients, nurses and chaplains.' *Clinical Nurse Specialist* 7, 4, 175–182.

Frankl, V.E. (1987) *Man's Search for Meaning: An Introduction to Logotherapy.* London: Hodder and Stoughton.

Harrison, J. and Burnard, P. (1993) *Spirituality and Nursing Practice.* Aldershot: Avebury.

McSherry, W. (1997) 'A descriptive survey of nurses' perceptions of spirituality and spiritual care.' Unpublished MPhil thesis, Hull: University of Hull.

Narayanasamy, A. (1991) *Spiritual Care: A Resource Guide.* Lancaster: Quay Books.

Oppenheim, A.N. (1992) *Questionnaire Design, Interviewing and Attitude Measurement*, new edn. London: Printer Publishers.

Shelly, J.A. and Fish, S. (1988) *Spiritual Care: The Nurse's Role*, 3rd edn. Illinois: Inter Varsity Press.

Waugh, L.A. (1992) 'Spiritual aspects of nursing: a descriptive study of nurses' perceptions.' Unpublished PhD thesis, Edinburgh: Queen Margaret College.

Subject Index

Page numbers in *italics* indicate figures, boxes and tables

Author Index

Page numbers in *italics* indicate figures, boxes and tables

Printed in Great Britain
by Amazon

35438991R00124